LIGHT, COLOR, AND ENVIRONMENT

A discussion of the Biological and Psychological Effects of Color, with Historical Data and Detailed Recommendations for the Use of Color in the Environment

FABER BIRREN

Revised Edition

VNR VAN NOSTRAND REINHOLD COMPANY

NEW YORK CINCINNATI TORONTO LONDON MELBOURNE

Revised edition first published in 1982
Copyright© 1969, 1982 by Van Nostrand Reinhold
Company Inc.
Library of Congress Catalog Card Number 76-102795
ISBN 0-442-21270-4

Printed in the United States of America

Van Nostrand Reinhold Company Inc.
135 West 50th Street, New York, NY 10020

Fleet Publishers
1410 Birchmount Road, Scarborough, Ontario M1P 2E7

Van Nostrand Reinhold Australia Pty. Ltd.
480 Latrobe Street, Melbourne, Victoria 3000

Van Nostrand Reinhold Company Ltd.
Molly Millars Lane, Wokingham, Berkshire, England
RG11 2PY

First edition published 1969 by Reinhold Publishing
Corporation

16 15 14 13 12 11 10 9 8 7 6 5 4 3 2

Contents

Introduction

Environment is a big and controversial subject these days. In his technological exertions man is accused of raising havoc with nature, and cries for action to be brought against him are heard.

The natural environment witnesses the pollution of water and air, and the despoiling of land. Factories, mills, power plants, smelters, strip miners are required by law to reduce if not cease their destructive effects. Fertilizers and insecticides upset nature's balance, killing defenseless birds and beasts. Public utilities are permitted to cut swathes through forests and to disenchant the eye with ugly transmission towers and substations. Nuclear power plants heat rivers to a near boiling point and thus deprive fish of their needed oxygen.

Again in the natural environment, man piles up mountains of chemical and radioactive waste. Waterways are contaminated with poisonous liquids, sewage, rubbish, garbage, at a rate that taxes human ingenuity in solving the problem of disposal. Man has even begun to proliferate the heavens with spent satellites, turning the space beyond the clouds into a semblance of a used car lot.

It is natural that an indignant essayist takes note of all this and begins to wonder indignantly where it will all end, what will become of us, and when man will come to his senses?

To be pragmatic, however, much of this diatribe is futile and directed into the wind. When prehistoric man first entered a cave and built a fire, he set himself in opposition against nature, and the battle between them has never ceased. Those who stand in awe of nature and see man as a demon may be overlooking or ignoring the fact that nature herself is at times quite an ogre. The spewing of a volcano can cause far more destruction than any man-made smelter. Floods, earthquakes, droughts, plagues, blights, show nature as the supreme devastator. If man is said to be arrogant and destructive before nature, mother nature is hardly a gentle or solicitous lover of man.

Man pollutes a river or a lake, is reprimanded (by himself), and tries his best to ameliorate the situation. In America, Lake Erie is slowly transforming into a swamp. Man's sewage may be in evidence, but nature, not man, is the one masterminding the project. It is nature who originally decided to make Lake Erie a swamp. She has made many swamps before. Hence, if man clears up his own pollution, what can he do to salvage nature's indiscretions?

Man strips forests and makes land barren. He can still show remorse. But what can be done when nature kills cedar trees in Bermuda and chestnut and elm trees in America? Who will be savior if not man?

Man can convert a desert, which nature has wrought by evolution, by irrigating it and making it thrive. Who is to be praised here?

The age-old dream of harmony between nature and man forever terminates in a conflict between the two. For his sins against nature man will have to do penance. But for his own survival man will have to be free of nature. He may respect the natural environment. But his own environment, his own cities, buildings, and abodes will have to withstand and control nature, if not be independent of her completely.

A scientist proclaims that if man continues to denude the land, he will deprive the atmosphere of oxygen and suffocate all humanity. (Threats of self-destruction through hydrogen bombs have lost appeal to most polemists.) Oxygen can be manufactured, however, from chemicals or sea water. The steel mills already pump oxygen scores of miles to their furnaces — and simultaneously act to reduce the smoke and soot produced.

Man can make his own oxygen. For that matter he can make his own food under artificial light and with fertilizers of his own concoction. With or without requesting the forgiveness of the gods, if man cannot live without nature entirely, he has assumed mastery over her so as not to fall victim to her callous mercy.

Virtually all human effort these days is leading toward the controlled environment. Urban centers grow larger, rural areas smaller. It is inconceivable that this trend can be stopped or reversed. Nature is being abandoned out in the country, where man has more or less allocated her realm. The cult of nature, the view of the mountains and the seashore, the babbling brook, the flower garden, the sunset and rainbow, are no longer the familiar habitats of man but tourist attractions for him to see and visit on weekends and holidays.

In the metropolis there is noticeably less longing for the wide open spaces. Even the artist has deserted nature for new and abstract expressions. He wants to become more intimate with man, to struggle and suffer along with him. He wants art to be bigger than ever in scale and to one day break into space itself. He endeavors to make art part of the environment, not something to be framed or set on a pedestal. Much of art will thus be more related to architecture, if not become an integral part of it.

The controlled environment is all too evidently here. Architects are visualizing underground and undersea communities — and aboveground cities completely enveloped by domes. All practical modes of transportation are air-conditioned; space travel would be impossible without it. Nature is still there, but man is insulating himself against her.

In a dynamic city like Montreal vast spaces exist below street level. There are subways, shops, restaurants, theaters, access to offices, hotels, apartment houses, railway terminals, garages. There is no need to venture outside, except to check on the transient state of nature's mood. Man is too busy these days to be discommoded by nature. He may be on the road to perdition, according to some dedicated obstructionists, but he is having quite an exciting time.

After all, it may be presumed that human ambitions need city life to find release. Pastoral regions are hardly conducive to achievements of any great quality or magnitude.

Environment is man's big challenge now and for the future. He must be safeguarded from his own worst enemy — himself. Out of doors he will be obliged to conserve nature's resources. Yet as he lives more and more unto himself, as the things he makes, builds, and destroys pile up about him as useless refuse, he will be forced to seek space for his wastes. He is already digging caves and wells, packing deadweight casks and hurling them into the sea. Nature will simply have to endure these desecrations and renounce some of her barren regions for those purposes. The more widespread the domains of man stretch out — usually from concentrated centers — the more nature will have to be pushed back. No conceivable retroversion can happen, for now the once rustic and pastoral man has left nature never again to return, except as a curious visitor.

Finally, the despoliation of beauty by the ugly structures of man built within his own bordered realms. What with control of air, heat, humidity, with food supply provided at will, what will be the appearance of the synthetic world he surveys? Man knows that if there are eternal laws of beauty they do not exist *out there* in nature but *here* within his own psyche. There is something born within him that demands equilibrium, rhythm, growth patterns, the parabolic curve — and color. It is not, as many suppose, that the root rectangle is harmonious in and of itself, or the rainbow, but that there is no beauty apart from the subject who sees it. If nature held secrets, she would be all beautiful. Maybe she is but man is a discriminating and selective soul, and he finds pleasure only in that which best suits his fancy.

There will be beauty in the controlled environment for the good reason that man will be able to make no excuses but to himself. His art forms will not be garnered from nature, for nature in an artificial world will herself look contrived. There will be security, health, survival. All that is about him will be his own doing, good or bad. He will not be at the mercy of primeval forces.

Perhaps on a Sunday he will go forth into nature by land, sea or air, gaze through the clear plastic shell of his conveyance and say to his children, "This may be hard to believe, but your ancestors used to live out there!"

CHAPTER ONE

The Vital Role of Perception

Color is a complex subject that can be studied from many points of view, each of which can be given specialized attention in books, technical courses, conferences, and seminars. Very often, experts in one field of color research may be quite indifferent to (or uninterested in) the studies of experts in other fields. Accumulated research is so extensive that no one scholar could possibly absorb or write coherently about all of it.

Color has physical, chemical, biological, physiological, optical, psychological, and neurological aspects; specialized areas of study include colorimetry and spectrophotometry, as well as the use of color in medicine, archaeology, anthropology, and art; colorblindness, color aptitude, chromatic adaptation, metamerism, and other major and minor matters are also areas of concern.

How much of this is relevant to architects or interior designers? To what extent should they become involved? It is doubtful whether artists (or architects) need to know the intricacies of color any more than good cooks need to know the chemical composition of the foodstuffs they use. Artistic and architectural expression commonly involves factors of creativity and innate feeling, which are hardly susceptible of material dissection.

This book takes a fairly simple and practical view. It is written for the architectural and interior-design community, and seldom has anyone from this group expressed much concern over spectrophotometry, chromatic adaptation, tristimulus specifications for color, or the psychophysics of color.

The reader should bear in mind that the word "color" refers to sensation. This may consist of radiant energy, wavelength, or vibration frequency; but, if the sun happens to strike an orchid in a tropic forest and no one is present to *see* the orchid, there is no color. Color is not the property of objects, spaces, and surfaces, as the ancients once supposed, but is merely a visual and neural interpretation of outer (and often inner) stimulation of the human visual process.

From the standpoint of physics, color is a form of electromagnetic energy that, in total, covers a wide span of phenomena. From short cosmic rays to atomic rays to x-rays to ultraviolet, visible, and infrared light to the microwaves of radio and TV, all have the same speed (about 186,000 miles per second) but wavelengths

vary from incredibly short frequencies to frequencies that are far apart from crest to crest.

How important are these variations? With short waves—those above visible light—for example, excessive exposure to ultraviolet energy can damage many materials such as plastics, cause fading, destroy plants, and be harmful to human beings. Yet a moderate amount of ultraviolet light is beneficial to living things.

Waves longer than those of visible light give more cause for worry. Reflective glass can reject the heat rays of the sun and cut down air-conditioning costs, yet infrared photography, known as thermography, can be used to make invisible heat rays visible. The army can use infrared equipment to spot animals—and enemies—in total darkness. Contours and secrets of the earth can be revealed. Buildings can be photographed to expose heat loss. Human afflictions can be diagnosed.

Lately much attention has been given to the inimical effects of microwaves. Restaurants, for example, may post signs stating that microwave ovens are used for cooking. Let anyone wearing a heart pacemaker beware! TV manufacturers are required to shield their sets against harmful radiation. Farmers, ranchers, and conservationists object to high-power transmission lines and microwave relay towers, charging that nature, plants, animals, and people are harmed by adverse radiation. A recent report maintained that the energy released by transmission towers atop one building of the World Trade Center may be injurious to tourists observing the city from the other building. A metal open screen may be required to ground the invisible transmission.

Architects and designers may also be concerned with the fact that excessive release of certain gases from the earth (due to aerosol sprays, exhausts of supersonic airplanes, or atomic tests) may use up the oxygen in the ozone layer above the earth and allow lethal rays from the sun to reach the earth.

Even visible light may be injurious. The laser, which uses visible light, often red light, has fantastic powers. It can drill holes in diamonds and steel and repair detached retinas in the human eye. It can cut cloth for tailors and saw lumber for carpenters. It may eventually guide missiles, knock holes in army tanks, and veer aircraft away from their flight patterns.

The laser, coupled with glass fibers as thin as or thinner than a human hair, can transmit innumerable sages simultaneously. Coupled with moving or stationary satellites above the earth, electronic beams are used to transmit data at will and from any place at any time. A recent RCA advertisement relates that the laser can transmit "the entire contents of a 24-volume encyclopedia in 3 minutes; 2500 phone conversations or 20 TV programs at the same time. Staggering amounts of information—all made to pass through a tiny thread of glass by a solid-state laser that radiates [visible] light from an area one-hundredth the size of the period at the end of this sentence."

Scientific measurement and specification of color follow what is known as the ICI (International Commission on Illumination) system. It accepts three primaries, red, green, and blue, and three light sources or illuminants, equivalent to daylight (C), sunlight (B), and incandescent light (A), under which color measurements may be made. Individual colors, from pure hue on the outer boundaries to white at the center, can be plotted.

As the system is involved with spectrophotometry, however, it is quite complex, and of doubtful benefit to architects and interior designers. Ralph M. Evans writes, in *An Introduction to Color*, that to make "really precise measurements" rigidly controlled conditions must exist. Otherwise, "Precise measurements under one set of conditions may be so far wrong when the conditions are changed that it is worse than a direct visual estimate." Alternative color-specification methods for architects are given in a later chapter of this book.

The value of colorimetry and spectrophotometry lies with those who make and sell raw materials and colorants, who have to meet strict standards of color uniform-

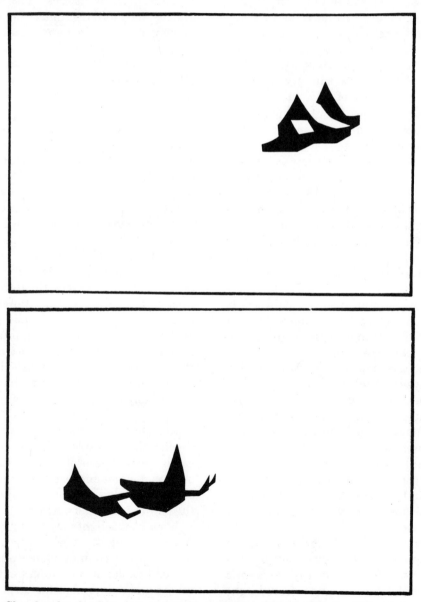

Sketches by the Canadian artist Marie Kohler, illustrating the difference between simple vision and complex perception.

ity from tone to tone, or who must be able to check the accuracy of *visual* color matches as they are repeated. The spectrophotometric chart can determine whether a color from one batch matches one from another—but it cannot correct errors or mismatches.

Well known to the physicist, but not always to the architect or interior designer, is the phenomenon of metamerism. Briefly stated, metameric colors may match under one light source but not under another. They occur primarily as a result of dyes, not of pigments. A run of carpeting, olive green under daylight, may appear brown under incandescent light. In order to avoid such problems, materials should be specified *after* viewing them under the light source to which they will be subjected. If lighting conditions are expected to vary (an interior lit by natural light during the day and artificial light at night, for example), the material should be examined under both illuminating conditions and accepted only if the results are acceptable.

Metamerism seldom causes trouble with paints or with most pigmented finishes or materials. While many architects insist on observing any and all colors under different light conditions, the fact that a color may appear yellowish when viewed in daylight under incandescent light is not necessarily due to metamerism. (All colors will change in this situation.) A metameric shift is unique and may reveal a startling change in hue from cool to warm or the reverse. The semiprecious gem alexandrite appears olive in daylight and ruby in candlelight.

A radical change of attitude, scientific and otherwise, regarding the human visual process has taken place in recent years, moving for the most part from optics, so to speak, to perception. It is naive today to speak of color sensation as a cameralike procedure that moves from the external world to the eye and up the optic nerve to the brain—or to accept the oft-repeated statement (quite untrue) that color perception depends on the light source that shines on or through it. The ingestion of LSD may suddenly expose a world of brilliant color that has its origin in the brain and is projected outward through the eye like a technicolor movie; no light source is involved. In a similar vein, Edwin D. Land (of Polaroid fame), through the use of projectors, filters, and light sources, has produced colors on a screen that were not related to a light source or filter. Color sensation truly exists in the brain. Energy transmitted from the outside world may indeed be a cause of much sensation but not a necessary cause.

Another phenomenon allied to perception is that of color constancy or chromatic adaptation. This involves the remarkable ability to see the world as normal under widely different conditions of light intensity or color quality. David Katz has made the intriguing statement that "The way in which we see the color of a surface is in large measure independent of the intensity and wavelength of the light it reflects, and at the same time definitely dependent upon the nature and intensity of the illumination in which it appears." A white surface (a card or a handkerchief) for example, viewed outdoors on a sunny day, will reflect many units of light. If the same white surface is then viewed in a dimly lit cellar, *it will still look white!* Colors are just as constant. If a white interior surface is pervaded by red (or yellow) incandescent light, it will still appear white. In fact, a white surface viewed under red illumination will look white even if it reflects more red than does an actual red surface lit by white light.

If this phenomenon remains somewhat bewildering, consider that many lighting demonstrations designed to illustrate the effects of different light sources (daylight, incandescent, cool fluorescent, warm fluorescent) on surface colors are specious—if they are confined to a relatively small shadow box. What is perceived in this situation may not prevail in larger, more active architectural spaces. Simply stated, chromatic adaptation ensures that a color will tend to appear normal under different conditions or tints of "white" illumination. In other words, if a person could go *inside* the compartments of a conventional light box, his or her vision would adapt accordingly: if he moved from a bluish to a yellowish, pinkish, or neutral illumination, he would notice scarcely any difference. The light box, due to its size, operates contrary to the actual facts of human perception.

The point, again, is that color effects must be analyzed and studied in their applicable environments. Technical considerations are less important than the evidence of vision. Color changes little with the chromatic quality of illumination, although, if tinted light sources are used, the appearance of human complexion must be checked carefully!

Let me make a final point about the relationship between form and color, referred to as physiognomic perception by some psychologists. This relationship emphasizes the active participation of the brain in the act and art of seeing. Leonardo da Vinci described the act of throwing a sponge soaked with color against a wall and seeing in the resulting abstract splotches all manner of things. It is natural to see objects and shapes in cloud formations, in rocks, in the silhouettes of hills and mountains. To all indications, the brain likes to make sense of what it sees. Mere vision may be passive in this regard, but perception is decidedly active.

Illustrated separately are two sketches in black and white by a Canadian artist, Marie Kohler, originally designed as Christmas cards, which express the difference between simple vision and more complex perception. If at first (or later) sight, one sees irregular black patterns on a white ground, this is simple vision. If there is a revelation of snow-covered farm buildings in a field of snow, this is perception. Architectural forms at times arouse unexpected responses. Houses seem to have eyes, nose, and mouth for windows; towers look like spiders; brown office buildings look like cakes.

CHAPTER TWO

The Primary Significance of Light

The four chapters that follow correlate the abundant data and information on the effects of color on living things. Virtually all of this stems from sources which the writer has patiently researched in the current scientific literature. Very little pure research has been undertaken by him, except for the analyses of case histories that have fallen within his personal experience. He is, thus, more of a technical scholar than a scientist. However, as a color consultant and writer on the subject, he has broadly applied the findings of pure research, being one of the relatively few men who have endeavored to avoid esthetics for an emphasis on the specific values that may be derived from the diligent inquiries and investigations of the true scientist.

Artificial, controlled environments have existed for a long time. Countless laboratory animals, mice, rats, guinea pigs, dogs, monkeys, animals in zoos, birds in aviaries, fish in aquariums have been reared under man-made conditions and often without exposure to natural light. How they have fared (including plants) will be remarked upon in later pages. Quite recently, and as will be duly noted, amazing facts have been discovered. The day is already here in which lighting for *biological purposes* will supplant or at least supplement lighting for mere purposes of vision. Further enlightenment has been enacted on the psychological effects of blank walls, boredom, and monotony. The ape can acquire neuroses and ulcers just as man can from the terrors of isolation. Not only is properly balanced light a prerequisite for all things, but the color of the light, the character of the environment, the stimulation of the senses (or lack of it) are all vital to normal life, as well as to survival itself.

Life may be said to begin with light and to be sustained by light. As man-made environments increase in size and extent, man-made light sources acquire great importance and demand new understanding and development.

The modern world, including man and all living things, has evolved, endured, and survived under the specific energy of sunlight. This solar energy pervades man's universe, provides man's food supply, and keeps man alive — along with other crawling, flying, and swimming creatures. Sunlight is balanced light, so to speak, emitting power that has a wide range in wavelength and frequency, each part or "octave" of which has a certain need and purpose.

The complete spectrum of electromagnetic energy, including sunlight, contains sixty or seventy "octaves." It begins, at one end, with radio waves of exceedingly great wavelength, proceeds through infrared rays, visible light, ultraviolet — the wavelengths becoming shorter — to reach its other extreme in X rays, gamma rays, and cosmic rays.

All this energy travels at the same rate of speed — about 186,000 miles a second — and differs in the length of waves as measured from crest to crest. Though mathematics of a rather fabulous order may be involved, measurements of the speed of light, of frequencies and wavelengths, are extremely accurate and are accepted throughout the scientific world.

The longest of all electromagnetic waves are employed for "wireless," high power transoceanic communication, ship-to-shore calling, direction finding, and the like. These waves may measure several thousand feet from crest to crest.

In the form of induction heat, long radio rays are employed in industry to raise the temperature of metals for hardening purposes in the period of a mere instant.

Commercial broadcasting rays fall next in order. Because they "bounce" back from the ionosphere of the sky, they will travel completely around the earth.

Next is the so-called "short-wave band," used for certain distance broadcasting, for police, ships, amateurs, and government.

Here also are the waves used in diathermy. By clamping electrodes to certain parts of the body, heat may be generated to relieve rheumatism, arthritis, neuralgia.

Next follow FM radio, television, radar, with the wavelengths becoming shorter and ranging from several meters to a fraction of a meter. This energy, however, penetrates the ionosphere and is not reflected back. It follows a straight path, requires rebroadcasting points, and may be sent out in controlled directions.

Next in order, long waves in the infrared region (invisible) have the power of penetrating distance and heavy atmosphere. Photographic plates sensitive to them are used to take pictures where the human eye has difficulty in seeing.

Radiant heat comes next as wavelengths shorten. Such energy is used for heating and drying purposes, and is emitted by steam radiators, electric heaters, and infrared lamps.

The sun's spectrum extends from the relatively long waves of infrared light, through the entire gamut of visible light (red, orange, yellow, green, blue, violet), into the shorter waves of ultraviolet light. At the red end are the ruby beams of the laser, which are today finding magical use. Laser beams have been bounced off the moon, have cut holes in diamonds, and healed detached human retinas. They are finding widespread use in communications, as cutting tools, and for three-dimensional photography (holography). They constitute one of the most remarkable and astonishing developments of modern science.

The longer waves of ultraviolet produce fluorescence in many substances.

Next follow the erythemal rays. This is the energy which produces suntan and which is employed for the synthetic production of vitamin D.

Still shorter ultraviolet energy has bactericidal properties. It is used to destroy certain microorganisms and for the sterilization of materials, water, and air.

On up the electromagnetic spectrum are the Grenz rays, or soft X rays, used therapeutically for many skin diseases. This energy does not have much power of penetration.

X rays of higher voltage and shorter frequency are used for diagnostic purposes and to treat certain forms of cancer.

Hard X rays, next in order, are used medically for deepseated afflictions — as well as to take radiographic pictures to detect flaws in metal.

Next follow the radium rays, discovered by Pierre and Marie Curie, and given therapeutic application in the early part of the twentieth century. They are used to cure many forms of cancer.

Toward the shortwave end of the electromagnetic spectrum are the emanations from nuclear fission, associated with the atom bomb and the bombardment of the atom nucleus. Such energy is rapidly finding its way into medicine.

Lastly, and of the shortest wavelengths, are the cosmic rays. Still a mystery, they probably are produced beyond the earth's atmosphere and spread their waves throughout the universe.

It is sunlight, however, real or artificial, that most concerns man's environment. Must it be balanced? Must it emit all energy from infrared through visible light to ultraviolet? What would happen to man if there were gaps?

The answers to these questions are not fully known. For example, if man were to build a community underground or undersea, light would have to be synthesized — but not merely for visual purposes! The light source would have to affect life itself, by demonstrating its effects upon absorption or acceptance by the eye of man and the tissues of his flesh.

There will have to be light to live by as well as to see by. That the problem of artificial light is no minor or incidental one is well confirmed by the fact that at a recent session (1967) of the International Commission on Illumination, the delegates agreed to a four-year study of the effects of light on "man who is often deprived of the natural dosage by virtue of his working and living environment."

To make one pertinent observation, where light may be needed for purposes other than vision, environments in which noncritical visual tasks are performed (recreation) may require higher levels than areas in which difficult eye tasks are performed (offices, schoolrooms)! This would largely reverse the present view of illuminating engineers.

To deal first with the general effects of light (and later with the effects of different colors), if man is to spend a good part of his time in artificial and controlled environments, he will have to construct his light sources with care. With plants, a common food source of man and beasts, the duration of sunlight and darkness is of primary importance. At the equator there are approximately twelve hours of sun and twelve hours of night each day. At the poles there may be twenty-four hours of sunlight in summer and twenty-four hours of darkness in winter, and intermediate latitudes range between these two extremes. These factors may, in part, account for the wide range of vegetation in the world.

Under the action of light, carbon dioxide and water are united in the presence of chlorophyll to form simple sugars. These sugars are elaborated into starch, proteins, organic acids, fats, and other products. Most of these compounds are foods for the plants, as well as for the animals that come to feed upon them. Further, the growth of plants is vitally affected by the length of day, the intensity of light, and by color even more than by temperature and moisture (which also depend on light).

It is imminent that some day there may be greenhouses without glass, and the science of phytoillumination, meaning the use of artificial light to aid plant growth, may predominate. Natural light is temperamental, but artificial light can easily be controlled. Such light will probably be dominant in red and blue, with green (which the plant doesn't seem to need) kept at a minimum to conserve electric power. There will be a peak in the visible red region of the spectrum where chlorophyll absorption is maximum.

As for lower animals, most living things not only react to light but are strangely sensitive to it. The lowly amoeba, for example, "sees" with its entire organism, moving or contracting itself as the light stimulus changes. Taken out of darkness, the amoeba may grow quiet. After a while, motion may be resumed until still another intensity strikes it. However, if the change of light is gradual rather than sudden, the amoeba may go about its simple business without much ado.

Certain species may have definite preferences for light intensity, moving about until a satisfactory brightness is found. Green hydras collect in relatively weak light; medusae collect in shaded regions; some polyps have a day-night rhythm. N. R. F. Maier and T. C. Schneirla write: "The place in which the animal finally settles is mainly determined by light, by the amount of oxygen in the water, and by the temperature. Except at extreme temperatures, or when the animal has been without food for some time, light is the most important factor."

Such creatures as worms are made uncomfortable by light, and some marine forms will move until they find darkness. Light from one direction will drive them in the opposite direction. General light overhead causes them to waver aimlessly. The earthworm, of course, fears light even more than it does the robin and will remain in nether regions until actually flooded out. Likewise, the cockroach scampers away from the light, while moths flutter toward it.

On up the scale, bird migration has been partially explained in terms of the length of day. As summer draws to an end and days grow shorter, a reaction takes place — possibly through the action of the pituitary gland — which speeds birds to more favorable climates. Migration may even take place before crops and seeds are ripe and before nature's autumn banquet is completely set.

In a series of fascinating experiments with birds, T. H. Bissonnette and others have proved that migration and sexual cycles are less dependent on temperature than on light. With the male starling, for instance, sexually quiescent during winter, testicle development occurred when the birds were given added light. As for starlings, Sol Zuckerman of England found that the starlings of Piccadilly Circus and Trafalgar Square in London — all exposed to brilliantly artificial light — had active reproductive organs at a time (during winter) when the starlings of Oxford were sexually impotent. One has cause to wonder if the great white ways of big cities are indeed not generators of physical appetite through the blaze of their lights and neon signs.

In other experiments the testes of immature ducks have been stimulated by light. Red wavelengths had the most active effect, while yellow and blue rays had little effect. Removal of light may cause anemia in some birds; whereas light will speed up blood count.

Changes in environmental lighting will affect gonad (sexual) activity in birds, as already stated. Richard J. Wurtman has much to report here. He mentions that Dutch and Japanese farmers have exposed song birds to extra illumination in autumn in order to induce singing — testicular activation being thus stimulated. This stimulation of sexuality in birds does not require light of high intensity; it can be well below that provided by sunlight. Here different wavelengths (colors) also hold significance, as mentioned above in the case of ducks.

To increase egg production in ducks and chickens, extra light is often used to supplement and extend the duration of daylight, particularly in winter. Researchers have found that as little as one footcandle of light is adequate for optimal egg production. R. J. Wurtman concludes, "Although relatively little information is available relating the intensity of light exposure to its efficacy as a neuroendocrine stimulus, it seems likely that the range in which intensity may be rate-limiting in mammals is well below that provided by the systems of artificial illumination generally in use."

Bissonnette found similar results with mammals. "Increased night lighting induces cottontail rabbits to undergo sexual activity in winter." In experiments with weasels, ferrets, and mink, he was able to achieve winter fur coloration during the hot days of midsummer. "It is, therefore, indicated that the assumption of white prime pelt by mink may be induced in summer in spite of relatively high temperatures or hastened in autumn by reducing the duration of the periods of light to which the animals are exposed daily."

Similar results were achieved with goats. Though a cow will give milk the year around, goats are less generous. Because they usually fail to breed between April and September, milk supply may be interrupted. Bissonnette has demonstrated that breeding, and consequently milk supply, can be controlled. "Results indicate that breeding cycles in goats are controlled by daily periods of light in such a way that short days induce breeding, while long days inhibit it."

As for mink, John Ott describes a case study in which mink were reared behind different colored plastic windows. Ordinarily, mink are quite vicious, particularly during the mating period. Mink kept behind *pink* plastic become increasingly aggressive and vicious. There was less frequency of pregnancy after mating. However, mink kept behind *blue* plastic became more docile and could be handled like house pets. All females became pregnant after mating. To draw an empirical conclusion, men as well as mink seem to be excited by red radiation and pacified by blue.

In Friedrich Ellinger's book, *Medical Radiation Biology*, many fascinating references are given on the influence of light on animals (and man). Length of daylight seems to be the most important of all features in stimulating sexual activity — or inhibiting it. Horses and donkeys reproduce during seasons of long daylight; there is a decrease in sexual activity from

October to January. When mares are exposed to additional illumination during winter months, ovarian activity may be affected. With cattle and sheep, fertility decreases during summer months, and this seems to be true also of pigs.

As for cows, one researcher in Alaska, W. J. Sweetman, "obtained an improvement in wintertime fertility by illuminating the animals 14 hours a day, whereas at this time of year daylight lasted from 6 to 8 hours." Another scientist, H. J. von Schumann "found that the number of hours of sunshine is the most important factor for the forming of horns" in stags. He assumed that light was absorbed through the hide of the deer, causing the formation of vitamin D and stimulating horn growth.

With animals (including man) it is apparent that light is vital to life. Some lower animals, frogs, and lizards have pineal organs underneath their skin which contain nerve cells similar to those found on the retinas of their eyes. These organs naturally respond to light. There is good evidence that radiant energy can actually penetrate into the mammalian brain. E. E. Brunt and associates caused light to penetrate the skulls of sheep, dogs, rabbits. They demonstrated "that light does reach the temporal lobes and hypothalmus in a variety of mammalian species." J. Benoit in experiments with ducks similarly reports that "a significant portion of visible radiations of higher wavelengths (essentially the red ones) can penetrate across the organs and tissues of the eye-window and reach the hypothalmus."

The hypothalmus, incidentally, is that part of the brain — at its base — which is believed to contain vital autonomic nerve centers and fibers which control such functions as respiration, heart action, digestion, etc. Where it is affected by light, the animal naturally responds in favorable or adverse ways depending on its needs. In an article for *Endrocrinology* (72: 962, 1963) W. F. Ganong and others reached the conclusion that "environmental light can penetrate the mammalion skull in sufficient amount to activate photoelectric cells imbedded in the brain tissue." This means that light is quite essential to a healthful and normal life and that nature has devised ways of having it affect the body through the tissues of the skin, the eyes, and even the skull itself.

Now as for human beings, H. L. Logan, a leading lighting engineer, has gathered data on the effects of light. Quoting his own experience and the research of others, Logan points out that light dilates the blood vessels, increases circulation, thus ridding the body of toxins and lightening the load on the kidneys.

Haemoglobin in the blood will be increased by light and decreased by darkness. Logan writes: "We are natural creatures originating in the subtropics, attuned to high levels of natural illumination. We can operate for less, for a penalty — poorer health, shorter life expectancy." And there are some hints that cancer and the rate of aging are somehow involved. Light also induces hormonal processes through the activation of endocrine glands.

It has been shown that sudden exposure to bright light stimulates the adrenal gland. There is, indeed, a time clock within all men which is regulated by day-night rhythms. As Richard J. Wurtman states, "These cycles synchronize a large number of biologic rhythms." The stimulation of light may come through the eyes, but it may also trigger effects through the skin and subcutaneous tissues. According to Wurtman, "It seems clear that light is the most important environmental input, after food, in controlling bodily function."

Sexual (gonad) activity in humans is quite related to light. Wurtman states, "The rather small amount of data available on different species [of animals] suggests that the absence of light induces gonad function in diurnally-active animals (e.g., humans, sheep), while the presence of light has this effect in nocturnal species (e.g., rat, ferret, raccoon, bat, cat)."

The whole matter is quite complex. Wurtman found, for example, that blind girls tended to reach an earlier first menstrual period and an earlier onset of puberty than girls with normal vision. He writes, "There is a possibility that light, acting on the neuroendocrine axis of the blind human . . . in the absence of retinal response to light, produces an imbalance which results in earlier menarche [menstrual function]."

However, among Eskimo women, menstruation may cease during the long arctic night, and the libido of Eskimo men may also be dormant. Here, in effect, lack of light would lead to a natural form of human hibernation. This is by no means a racial characteristic individual to Eskimos. The same effects seem to occur to any persons exposed to alternately long periods of sunlight and darkness. With the onset of the long arctic winter, human sexual desire fails. It is revived again with the dawn of spring. Girls of the tribes of North Greenland may marry at fourteen or fifteen, but menstruation may not occur until they reach nineteen or twenty. (The paradox here is that, in Wurtman's study quoted above, blind girls in temperate zones tended to reach an early menstrual function.) Eskimo children, because of all this, are generally born nine months after the advent of spring and the return of the arctic sun.

John Ott, who has undertaken a remarkable body of work on light and color, concurs with Logan. "Life on this earth has developed in response to the full spectrum of natural sunlight, and variations in the wavelength distribution by artificial light sources, or distortion of the wavelength distribution of sunlight filtered through glass, seems to result in variations for normal growth development in both plants and animals."

Ott hints about cancer as well. He recommends the use of contact lenses which transmit the full ultraviolet spectrum.

Man's worship of the sun and his need for energy will have to be respected in the controlled environment. Heliotherapy is perhaps as old as civilization. In his excellent book, *The Biologic Fundamentals of Radiation Therapy*, Friedrich Ellinger writes:

Knowledge of the therapeutic action of light is one of mankind's oldest intellectual possessions. The earliest experiences depended of course upon nature's own light source, the sun. Sun-bathing was practiced even long ago by the Assyrians, Babylonians and Egyptians. A highly developed sun- and air-bathing cult existed in ancient Greece and Rome. The old Germans regarded the healing power of sunlight very highly and worshipped the rising sun as a deity. The Incas of South America also practiced a sun cult.

However, the sun worshipers, together with the alchemists and mystics, lost prestige after the Middle Ages. Though there were a few obscure champions from time to time, it was not until the nineteenth century that heliotherapy was again recognized.

The pioneer of light research was Niels R. Finsen of Denmark. In his early years he held a strong interest in color and believed in the treatment of smallpox with visible red light to prevent scar formation. Later (1896) he wrote of the actinic properties of sunlight and founded a Light Institute for the cure of tuberculosis. He was awarded a Nobel prize in 1903 and later reported startling cures among some 2,000 patients, using both sunlight and artificial ultraviolet light.

Credit is also due Downs and Blunt of England, who, in 1877, discovered the bactericidal action of ultraviolet radiation. This gave full evidence that sunburn was not produced by heat rays alone and that in waves of higher frequency than visible light, science had a great therapeutic medium.

There are two interesting observations to be noted regarding sunlight and human life. In India, rickets is a common affliction among higher caste Hindus, no doubt because the religious system requires mothers and children to dwell in complete indoor isolation. Hence, because the body is deprived of sunlight, it suffers from vitamin D deficiency.

Ultraviolet radiation is essential to human welfare. It prevents rickets, keeps the skin in a healthy condition, is responsible for the production of vitamin D, destroys germs, and affects certain necessary chemical changes in the body. It is used in the treatment of certain skin diseases, in erysipelas, and in skin tuberculosis. In indoor aquariums some virus diseases can be cured by exposing fish to a moderate amount of ultraviolet. Equally good results have been achieved among reptiles, birds, and other animals.

It may be employed to irradiate foodstuffs such as lard, oil, and milk to form vitamin D. Curiously, however, cod-liver oil loses its better properties after irradiation. Although ordinary window glass and many materials will absorb it, ultraviolet light is effectively scattered by the atmosphere, and its benefits are found even in smoky cities.

After exposure to ultraviolet, human skin becomes pigmented. A tanned complexion is perhaps nature's method of building up protection, even though protection against ultraviolet is often achieved without pigmentation.

Yet a glowing tan is by no means a sign of vigorous health. Overexposure to sunlight may make the complexion wrinkled and old in time. More seriously, Blum points out that prolonged exposure to sunlight "may stimulate the production of malignant tumors of the skin." Apparently the old adage of moderation in all things must include the beach and the sun deck.

John Ott believes in a "theory of the importance of the full spectrum of sunlight energy." He refers to the potency of daylight in the health of virtually all living things. Of human ills, he writes: "Some doctors have said cancer is a virus or at least is in some way associated with it. If this is so, then the possibilities of influencing body chemistry by the characteristics of the light energy received through the eye might conceivably be an important factor in the metabolism of the individual cells of the tissues of the body."

To speak further of ultraviolet energy, the artificial environment will no doubt find need for it, but in moderate amount. Discovery of the antirachitic action of ultraviolet was made by K. Huldschinsky in 1919, and this led in time to the photochemical formation of vitamin D. When the body is exposed to ultraviolet rays, there is dilation of the capillaries of the skin. Blood pressure falls slightly. In addition to a feeling of well being, there is a quickening of pulse rate and appetite, plus a stimulation of energy. What happens is that the brain is caused "to function on a level of higher activity." As Ellinger writes, "The laboratory experiences on the effect of ultraviolet irradiation on physical fitness have been confirmed by performance studies on workmen, sportsmen and school children." Work output can actually be increased, a fact that will be mentioned again later in the chapter on biological lighting.

Ultraviolet radiation tends to increase protein metabolism. It will thus help to reduce sugar level in the blood of diabetics — having an effect similar to that of insulin.

Of waves longer than visible light (infrared), there is little to be told. Such energy obviously produces heat within the human body — as do the still longer radio rays of diathermy. Harold F. Blum in his remarkable book, *Photodynamic Action and Diseases Caused by Light*, remarks that "it cannot be assumed this part of the spectrum [infrared] is very active biologically."

However, the heating effect of invisible rays at the red end of the spectrum is known to everyone who has ever used a hot water bottle.

Infrared rays are also thought to weaken the bactericidal action of ultraviolet rays. They also seem to destroy the antirachitic effect of vitamin D. While such "heat" rays may be generally beneficial, they represent a great hazard to the human eye. While ultraviolet waves are strongly absorbed by the eye media, infrared waves are not. The latter may be responsible for the development of cataracts. Ellinger writes, "On the basis of animal experiments, A. Vogt believes that cataracts in workers exposed to fire (welders, glass blowers, etc.) are due to the action of infrared rays."

Living things on earth have been conditioned to solar radiation through countless ages. Had this energy been different, no doubt the world — and man — would have been different (had they existed at all). Because solar radiation is predominant in rays of light visible to the human eye, with added shorter waves in ultraviolet and added longer waves in infrared, these frequencies must be vital to animal life (and to plants) and must influence it accordingly.

Perhaps it won't be easy, but if man hazards extermination through lack of oxygen, atomic radiation, water and air pollution, the disruption of nature, he also may find himself in trouble if he does not comprehend the secrets of sunlight and adapt them to his purpose in the establishment of his environments.

Further remarks on light and illumination as related to health, visibility, seeing comfort, and human appearance will be found in chapters that follow.

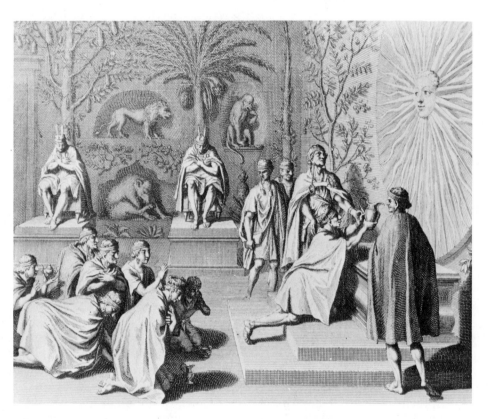

Worship of the sun by the Incas of South America, from an 18th-century engraving.

CHAPTER THREE

The Biological Effects of Color

Let the emphasis now be shifted from the effects of light in general to the effects of different colors or hues. Plants thrive mostly on the visible (to humans) wavelengths of sunlight and may be inhibited or destroyed if exposed solely to infrared or ultraviolet. Men and plants, of course, have gone through life together. Yet in modern medical practice therapeutic effects for *visible* colors are disregarded more or less for the healing qualities of *invisible* infrared and ultraviolet!

Much research is now being conducted on the effects of light and color on plants, with considerable influence on horticulture. Among prominent investigators in the field are H. A. Borthwick of the U.S. Department of Agriculture, Stuart Dunn of the University of New Hampshire, and R. van der Veen and G. Meijer of the Philips Research Laboratories in Holland (to mention but a few). It was Borthwick who noted an antagonism between visible red light and invisible infrared. Red would cause lettuce seed to sprout, for example, while infrared would put the sprouts back to sleep. Similarly, red would inhibit flowering of short-day plants and promote flowering of long-day plants. R. van der Veen and G. Meijer reported that there was maximum absorption of red light and hence maximum plant action. Blue also has its effects, but yellow and green are neutral or reduce activity, and short ultraviolet will destroy the plant. What is unusual is that plants seem most responsive to red and blue, and inactive to yellow and yellow-green. However, the human eye finds maximum sensitivity (visibility) to yellow and yellow-green. In handling plants in a greenhouse under artificial light, weak green illumination is "safe light," for there is little, if any, plant response to it. "This safe light is to the plant physiologist what the ruby light was for the photographer."

Stuart Dunn's findings in growing tomato seedlings are particularly interesting. "The yield produced by the Warm White lamps was highest of all the commercially available fluorescent lamps. Next to it stood that of the Blue and Pink lamps. Green and Red were low. The experimental 'high intensity' red lamps produced the highest yield of all." (Sylvania Lighting Products, by the way, manufactures a "Gro-Lux" fluorescent lamp for phytoillumination.) "Stem growth (elongation) is promoted especially by the yellow part

of the spectrum." However, "Succulence is increased by the long wavelengths (red) and decreased by blue light."

Growing flowering plants completely under artificial light is fast becoming a national hobby. And as it does, the mystery and magic of color become more impressive.

John Ott's work with colored light and plants holds great fascination. Applying controlled light sources as well as daylight, he has encountered several weird phenomena. Chrysanthemums can be made to flower any month of the year by regulating their exposure to light, cutting it off in the long days of summer, or lengthening the short days of winter with extra hours of artificial illumination. This practice is now universally used by florists in greenhouse cultivation of chrysanthemums and poinsettias. According to Ott, blue light and filters caused morning glory buds to open. When the light source was "warm" in nature, buds tended to collapse and shrivel. Ott writes, "It is the specific band of wavelengths at the red end of the spectrum that were the controlling factor in preventing the morning glory buds from opening normally."

With the pumpkin, which has separate male and female flowers. Ott discovered quite by accident that regular fluorescent light withered the female flowers but not the male. When bluish daylight fluorescent tubes were employed, the reverse happened, the male flowers withered and the female blossomed. As Ott writes, "The fact that either male or female flowers can be brought forth by controlling slight variations in color or more length of light, opens up some interesting possibilities for investigation."

Color vision is not apparent in the lowest forms of animal life. It does exist in insects, fish, reptiles, and birds, and though lacking in most mammals, is present in apes and men.

Insects' color vision differs from that of men. Scientists are largely agreed that the eye of the insect responds to the yellow region of the spectrum (but not the red) and is sensitive to green, blue, violet, up to ultraviolet. In experimenting with fruit flies, E. N. Grieswood noted a reaction to wavelengths invisible to man, which in shortness of frequency approached X rays. In similar tests, L. M. Bertholf found the range of sensitivity in bees extends from about 550 millimicrons (yellow-green), through green, blue, violet and into waves as short as 250 millimicrons (ultraviolet). The human eye is sensitive to a region extending from about 700 millimicrons to 400.

Insects show definite color "preferences." Ants placed in a box illuminated by a complete spectrum of sunlight will carry their larvae (always kept in darkness) out of the ultraviolet and into the visible red. Von Frish has demonstrated that bees can be made to see the difference between a blue and a gray of the same brightness, and can also differentiate blue from violet or purple, and yellow from any of these. This has been demonstrated by training bees to fly to certain colors to obtain food. The bee is hopelessly confused by red and cannot differentiate it from neutral gray targets. H. Molitor found that when wasps enter a nest, they prefer a black entrance to a blue one, and blue to red. Red seems to interfere with the normal growth of cockroaches. The Oriental peach moth, when given a choice, is most responsive to blue and violet. With silkworms, violet light is active and red light inactive. A group of researchers (H. B. Weiss, F. A. Soroci, E. E. McCoy, Jr.) in testing about 4,500 insects, mostly beetles, found that seventy-two percent reacted positively to some wavelength: thirty-three percent to yellow-green, fourteen percent to violet-blue, eleven percent to blue, and eleven percent to ultraviolet. Few showed any attraction to warm colors. "It thus appears that in general the shorter wavelengths of light are more stimulating and attractive, whereas the longer wavelengths are considerably less stimulative and perhaps repellent in nature to coleopterous (beetles) forms of life."

Though color in the life of fish is far less significant than brightness, form, and motion, G. L. Walls points out that "No fish is known *not* to have color vision." Scientific work on color vision is plentiful. R. Hess determined that fish see green as the lightest color, then blue, yellow, orange, with red the darkest color of all. "The intensity of any color needed to balance pure yellow was only half that required to balance green." According to Walls, "Fishes generally seem either to shun red, or to prefer it decidedly." This may be due, in part, to the fact that red radiation is quickly absorbed as it passes through water and is, therefore, not a common experience for fish. In experiments with mud minnows, Cora Reeves found that respiration rate rose with the increase of brightness. When ruby glass was placed across an artificial light source, respiration rate increased even more. "In this experiment it was perfectly clear that the response was to redness as such, since the respiration rose with an increase of brightness, but rose still higher when that brightness was somewhat reduced by a filter which introduced hue" [Walls].

The influence of color on the behavior of fish has been proved by experiments such as these. Working with flounders, S. O. Mast painted the floors of tanks in various hues. Where a fish had been blue-adapted, it tended to choose this color as a resting place and to avoid other hues. In experiments with tropical fish, Ott studied the effects of different wavelengths and intensities. The young produced under pinkish fluorescent light resulted in eighty percent female and twenty percent male. No young were produced under bluish fluorescent light.

Even feeble amounts of light will affect the normal development of fish. According to Ott, "When the death rate among brook trout eggs at the New York State Hatchery, Cold Spring, suddenly shot up to the ninety percent bracket from under ten percent . . . Dr. Alfred Perlmutter of New York University traced the cause to installation of new forty-watt fluorescent lights in the ceiling. Another investigator, working with rainbow trout, found that the violet and blue components of white or visible light are more deadly than the green, yellow and orange bands."

Fish capable of color change depend upon visual processes and lack the ability when blinded. Here again there is a curious disregard of brightness alone. Except under extremely high or low illumination, fish will not respond to gradual changes in the amount of light entering its eye. Yet the moment its substrate or background is modified in lightness or darkness, the skin of the fish will rapidly conform in "value" to it.

A turtle's ability to find water will perhaps always remain a mystery. Theories are many. One is that the turtle avoids shadow, knowing instinctively that clear reaches of sky are without overhanging verdure and therefore must have water underneath. Another theory is that blue is the attracting force. Certainly orientation to the sun is meaningless, for turtles will persistently move in any direction that is clear and unobstructed; and color may be the clue. In turtles, as in other reptiles, color vision is well developed. While discrimination of brightness and intensity is poor, colors are readily distinguished from grays. According to Walls, "The most important hues for the turtle appear to be orange, green and violet. Yellow and yellow-green, when not accurately discriminated, were apparently most often seen as orange; but red was separated from the general orange category and seemed to be more akin to violet for the animal, which thus had a closed color circle." Wagner, in studies of lizards, noted discrimination of red, orange, yellow, yellow-green, ice blue, deep blue, and violet. Vision was keenest to red and blue, and weakest to green.

The previous chapter has made reference to the effects of light and color on birds. Response to color reaches a high development in birds. Here the organs of sight are intricate and versatile. Many birds, for example, have two foveal areas on their retinas, enabling them to see sharply while feeding as well as in flight. The eyes of birds also contain colored droplets (red, orange, and yellow), and the predominating yellow droplets in most diurnal birds are a definite aid to vision. They cut out blue light, minimize glare and dazzle, and, according to Walls, let through, "unimpeded, most of nature's hues." Similarly, the red droplets aid the bird during early morning feeding when the sun's rays, slanting through space, are reddish in tint. The kingfisher (also the turtle) has a predominance of red droplets which unquestionably aid vision in glaring water. Perhaps for the above reason, most birds are partially blind to blue and see red colors with remarkable clarity.

Color preference among birds is definite and seems to be associated with their feeding habits. Hummingbirds favor red and will feed more readily from red vials or containers. In *The Color of Life*, Arthur G. Abbott points out the disinterest of birds in the color green. Because rodents are color-blind, poisons meant to destroy field mice and rodents can be dyed green so that birds will not touch them. As Abbott reports, where poisoned seeds were uncolored, many birds died, but where the poisoned seeds were green, the birds refused them. The field mice were destroyed, color or no color.

Recently the British have considered the coloring of airfields to drive away birds which are a hazard to planes. Purple seems to be the best repellent, and experiments are being conducted with dyed grass or the hybrid creation of purple grass itself.

Because most mammals are virtually color-blind, their reactions to color are all the more interesting. Rodents kept under blue light have had the same growth rate as those reared under normal light. Under pink or red light, however, appetite has been increased and weight accelerated. Yet prolonged exposure of mice to pink illumination has resulted in death (see Chapter 6).

In experiments with mice, John Ott kept over 1,000 in separate colonies under three conditions: bluish fluorescent light, pinkish fluorescent light, and natural daylight. Here were some of the results. The colony under natural daylight produced 50 percent females and 50 percent males. The colony under bluish fluorescent light produced 70 percent females and about 30 percent males. The colony under pinkish fluorescent light produced about 30 percent females and 70 percent males. Despite tradition, it would seem that blue is for girls and pink for boys.

In a study performed for the U.S. Atomic Energy Commission (1968) three researchers, Spalding, Archuleta, and Holland, investigated the influence of visible colors on voluntary activity in albino RF strain mice. The rodents were placed in cubicles for periods of 18 hours, rested, and then placed for 18 hours in other cubicles until all environments were tested. The measure of activity was determined by the revolutions of activity wheels (like those seen in squirrel cages).

Mice are nocturnal animals and hence most active in darkness. The test resulted in these findings: there was most activity in darkness; next greatest activity was with red. (The RF strain mouse experiences red as darkness.) "Activity in yellow light was significantly greater than in daylight, green, blue, and significantly less than in dark and red." Incidentally, blind mice showed little difference in activity, regardless of color, bearing out that the effects discovered were "due to visual receptors."

Again, according to Ott, breeders of chinchillas will have a relatively high percentage of males if the animals are kept under ordinary (warm) incandescent light, and a correspondingly high ratio of females if kept under daylight (bluish) incandescent illumination. The use of bluish artificial light now has become common practice among commercial breeders of chinchillas. Maybe the eternal problem of sex preference in babies will one day be solved through the medium of colored light. At the moment, it would seem that kings who desire male heirs would do well to light the boudoir with pink bulbs.

Animal life which lives directly and indirectly on plant food is definitely responsive to visible light. Lowly organisms will orient to it, at times responding throughout the entire body. As long ago as 1900, Oscar Raab noted the toxicity of dyes on microscopic organisms. A gelatinous creature might move in and out of intense sunlight and be literally at home. Yet with an inert dye introduced, it could be sensitized and destroyed because of excessive light absorption. Although the damaging energy might be due in large part to ultraviolet, such metabolic effects have also been traced to visible light as well.

Most persons are familiar with such evidences of light sensitivity in human beings. Skin eruptions may follow exposure to sunlight after the use of cosmetics and ointments. "Strawberry rash" and "buckwheat rash" may be traced to light sensitivity brought about by eating certain foods. Here again, while ultraviolet may be the cause of irritation, visible light may be involved. In some rare forms of urticaria solare, visible blue and violet light (with ultraviolet and infrared excluded) has been found to cause an erythema attended by discoloration and swelling.

In fact, the medical profession has recently been impressed by the discovery of A. Kilner, that visible light may reverse or arrest the injurious effects of ultraviolet light. Two further investigators, Rieck and Carlson, have shown that the death rate in albino mice, brought about by severe exposure to ultraviolet, may be substantially reduced where visible light is used as a palliative.

It seems apparent that human beings, like all other living things, have a radiation sense. What is significant is that such sense may be independent of conscious vision itself. Awareness of the existence of light will be noted by completely blind individuals, even where heat and ultraviolet energy are excluded. Some authorities are of the opinion that the visible light of the sun acts directly on the superficial layers of the skin and has definite metabolic effects.

No matter, reactions to color through the eye itself are many, varied, and intriguing. In the main, color effects tend to be in two directions — toward red and toward blue — with the yellow or yellow-green region of the spectrum more or less neutral. Further, these two major colors induce different levels of activation both in the autonomic nervous system and in the brain.

Red seems to have an exciting influence. Kurt Goldstein writes, "It is probably not a false statement if we say that a specific color stimulation is accompanied by a specific response pattern of the entire organism." With reference to red, he mentions the case of a woman with a cerebellar disease who had a tendency to fall unexpectedly. When she wore a red dress such symptoms were more pronounced. Goldstein points out that tremor, torticollis, and some conditions of Parkinsonism "can at times be diminished in severity if the individuals are protected against red or yellow, if they wear, for instance, spectacles with green lenses."

Working with infants, who obviously had no prior experience with color, Josephine M. Smith noted that blue light tended to lessen activity and crying. It may be that man's reactions to color in later life are not due solely to cultural training (many psychologists have assumed this), but to deeper-lying responses. Differential responses to color have also been observed in blindfolded subjects. This would again suggest that human reactions to color, while influenced by consciousness, are not altogether dependent on it.

There is a general light tonus in the muscular reactions of the human body. Conditions of muscular tension and relaxation are noticeable and measurable as tonus changes. Mostly they rise from complete inaction and are more active with warm colors than with cool ones.

Through optic excitation, A. Metzger observed that when light was directed on one eye of many animals and humans, a tonus condition could be produced in the corresponding half of the body. Accompanying these tonus changes were changes in "the superficial and deep-seated sensations, both showing a regular dependence upon optical stimuli." He concluded that the influence of light not only acted on the muscles but was effective in producing changes over the entire organism.

As for experimental method, Metzger had his subject stretch out his arms horizontally in front of his body. When light was thrown on one eye, there would be a tonus increase on the same side of the body. The arm on the side of the light would raise itself and deviate toward the side of the illumination. When colors were employed, red light would cause the arms to spread away from each other. Green light would cause them to approach each other in a series of jerky motions. In cases of torticollis, exposure to red light increased restlessness, while green light decreased it.

In similar experiments described by Felix Deutsch and Friedrich Ellinger, it was found (by H. Ehrenwald) that when the face and neck are illuminated from the side, the outstretched arms will deviate toward the light if red and away from it if blue. To quote Deutsch, "This reaction takes place also when the eyes are tightly sealed to exclude light."

Goldstein who has worked extensively with color and written much about it concludes:

The stronger deviation of the arms in red stimulation corresponds to the experience of being disrupted, thrown out, abnormally attracted to the outerworld. It is only another expression of the patient's feeling of obtrusion, aggression, excitation, by red. The diminution of the deviation [to green illumination] corresponds to the withdrawal from the outer world and retreat to his own quietness, his center. The inner experiences represent the psychological aspect of the reactions of the organism. We are faced in the observable phenomena with the physical aspect.

Goldstein also noted that judgment could be affected by color. Time, for example, was likely to be overestimated under red light and underestimated under green or blue light.

Not all investigations have been able to verify such reactions as arm deviation, but the majority have confirmed the fact that there is marked activation with color. Fere in competent experiments showed autonomic arousal and increased muscular pressure for all colors, green causing the least increase and red the most.

Light and color undoubtedly affect body functions, just as they exert an influence over so-called mind and emotion. In what is known as the unity of the senses, individual experiences are seldom confined to one organ or a sense of the organism. As Sherrington concludes, "All parts of the nervous system are connected together and no part of it is probably ever capable of reaction without affecting and being affected by the other parts, and it is a system certainly never absolutely at rest."

Gestalt psychologists such as Heinz Werner have reviewed phenomena in which sounds will affect color perception. Kravkov, Allen, and Schwartz have found that loud noises, strong odors and tastes, tend to raise the sensitivity of the eye to green and to decrease sensitivity to red.

Thus all experiences, color included, have definite interrelationships. Specifically in reference to color, however, here are the words of Deutsch. "Every action of light has in its influence physical as well as psychic components." All persons are aware of "sensations and psychic excitations, which through the vegetative nervous system, boost all life functions: increase the appetite, stimulate circulation, etc., and through these manifestations the physical influence of light upon the disease process is in turn enhanced."

It may thus be generalized that color affects muscular tension, cortical activation (brain waves), heart rate, respiration, and other functions of the autonomic nervous system — and certainly that it arouses definite emotional and esthetic reactions, likes and dislikes, pleasant and unpleasant associations. Research to date, however, has lacked good scientific control. Some tests have been largely empirical, and others have been concerned with certain human functions only.

A later chapter will deal with psychological reactions to color. At this point in the book there is a good opportunity to build links between physiological and neural responses to color and the emotional interpretations that so often follow.

In a remarkable book by Barbara B. Brown, *New Mind, New Body*, this statement is made: "The skin sees in technicolor." It is "also a good detector and seems to reflect the way in which brain neurons process color information. Experiments demonstrating body reactions to color support the common belief that colors induce emotional states which are specific to different hues."

Dr. Brown is Chief of Experimental Physiology at the Veterans Administration Hospital in Sepulveda, California. She also lectures in the Department of Psychiatry at the UCLA Medical Center and has pioneered in biofeedback research. According to Dr. Brown, the polygraph (lie detector) measures such physiological reactions as heart action, respiration, and skin response (to perspiration). The electroencephalograph (EEG) similarly measures brain waves. In general, there is a high response to colors such as red and orange, and a lower response to green and blue—quite apart from what a person might "think" or "feel" about color.

Dr. Brown sought to determine "whether feelings about color modify brain waves or whether brain waves are first affected by colors and the feelings developed later." There is a definite connection between physical and emotional reactions to color. Dr. Brown concludes that "the overlap between the associations between color and brain waves . . . suggests the possibility that subjective activity relating to colors may originate from the same underlying neuronal processes as do the brain waves . . . I tend to favor the concept that the brain cell, neuronal response to color came first, since in my studies and those of others the brain electrical response to red is one of alerting or arousal, whereas the brain electrical response to blue is one of relaxation. This happens in animals as well as man."

This would settle the debate over the primacy of aesthetics or biology; in terms of color, they go together.

CHAPTER FOUR

Vision — a Dynamic Process

Vision does not obey the simple laws of optics. Although the optical system of the human eye is far from perfect, nature has performed miracles designing the retina and cortical system of vision.

"Structurally, the retina may be regarded as a light-sensitive expansion of the brain," W. D. Wright has said. It is the photosensitive lining at the back of the eyeball, within which physical light produces nervous impulses that are forwarded to the brain. The human retina has two types of photoreceptor cells, the rods, (about one hundred thirty million in each eye) distributed rather uniformly over its entire expanse, and the cones (about seven million), especially numerous and confined in the central area and fovea of the retina.

Although the exact process of vision is still a mystery, science generally approves the so-called "duplicity theory," first stated by Max Schultz in 1866. This theory states that low-intensity vision is a function of the rods of the retina, and high-intensity vision is a function of the cones. The rods, it is believed, react chiefly to brightness and motion in subdued light. The cones react to brightness and motion but also to colors. Accordingly in the central fovea and in the region next to it, most of the action of seeing takes place; for only here does the eye perceive fine detail and color. Foveal sight is essentially cone vision and day vision; peripheral sight is rod vision, especially useful at night.

Quite recently Edwin H. Land has presented a new "retinex theory" of color vision, to be described later, in which greater importance is attached to reactions to brightness than to colors themselves.

The foveal area of the retina is permeated by a yellowish pigment (the so-called "maculalutea" or yellow spot). Although this tiny area measures less than one-sixteenth of an inch in diameter, it is crowded with tens of thousands of photoreceptors, especially the cones, *each* of which is thought to have its own connection to the brain. Hence, there is good reason for the fovea to be remarkably sensitive to fine detail. In the periphery, however, nerve connections to the cones and rods are arranged in groups. Wright observes, "This in turn implies that the peripheral retina is quite incapable of resolving fine detail in an image, although at the same time it enables the response

from weak stimuli to be summated and gives the periphery an advantage over the fovea in the detection of faint images."

The cortical region of the human brain responsible for sight has areas corresponding to the fovea and periphery of the eye, with one interesting difference: the area devoted to peripheral vision is relatively small; the area devoted to foveal vision is relatively large. In effect, this means that while the fovea is little more than a dot on the retina, its function in responding to fine detail and color is extremely vital and requires a sizable bit of "gray matter." Conversely, while the extrafoveal periphery of the retina is relatively large, its simpler response to brightness, motion, and crude form needs less area within the brain.

That vision is as much in the brain as it is in the eye is well demonstrated by a few more oddities. Human eyes see better than the eyes of lower animals because human brains are superior. Stimuli received by any eye, in fact, have no particular meaning until the brain interprets them. A rudimentary eye bud can be taken from a hen's egg and made to grow in a salt solution. It will actually develop and form a lens. Without a brain connection, however, it does not "see."

Human eyes are not the most complex or highly developed in nature. As R. L. Gregory states, "Complicated eyes often go with simple brains." The visual acuity of the hawk, for example, is four times superior to that of man.

James P. C. Southall writes in *Introduction to Physiological Optics*:

If the eye has had no previous experience to guide it in some particular instance, it may be difficult for the brain to interpret the visual phenomenon correctly. If therefore the chain of communication between the central part of the organ of sight and the adjacent optical memory tract is impaired or entirely broken in one of its links, the external object may indeed be visible to the eye but it cannot be comprehended by the brain. Under such circumstances the spectator will see it *per se* and indeed may perhaps even be able to draw a sketch of its outlines, but he cannot call it by name or make out what it signifies, unless he can also touch it and reinforce his sense of sight by the aid of other senses.

In short, seeing is not a matter of recording external stimuli alone, but of bringing forth mental recollections and experiences.

Southall further writes:

Good and reliable eyesight is a faculty that is acquired only by a long process of training, practice and experience. Adult vision is the result of an accumulation of observations and associations of ideas of all sorts and is therefore quite different from the untutored vision of an infant who has not yet learned to focus and adjust his eyes and to interpret correctly what he sees. Much of our young lives is unconsciously spent in obtaining and coordinating a vast amount of data about our environment, and each of us has to learn to use his eyes to see just as he has to learn to use his legs to walk and his tongue to talk.

In man's binocular vision, the foveal area of the retina will simultaneously focus form, brightness, color, and detail, assuring a clear image and a perfect sense of size, shape, and distance. At the same time, the retina's peripheral areas will respond to brightness change or motion on the outer boundaries of the field of vision. The baseball player, with his fovea on the ball, will use his periphery to guide the arc of his bat, and the prizefighter, with his eye on his opponent's chin, will be protected from "haymakers" coming in from the sides.

The human equation operates as well in discriminating detail. Ralph M. Evans writes, "A telephone wire may be seen at a distance greater than a quarter of a mile." Under the best of conditions an image so small could hardly be recorded by a glass lens and photographic plate, but the human eye and brain are able to construct a remarkably accurate image. Apparently, the retina requires only a few hints of the existence of the wire, whereupon the brain pieces it together.

In speed of seeing, the brain records a fairly clear image of a scene or object, though the exposure may be a mere fraction of a second. Flashes of light will produce higher subjective brightness than light shone continuously. When two lights are flashed simultaneously, one striking the fovea and the other the periphery of the retina, the light seen foveally will appear to flash ahead of the other. Similarly, blue lights require a slower blinking rate than red lights, if such blinking is to be seen. In his *The Vertebrate Eye*, G. L. Walls states: "A Swedish railroad recently found that certain red signals, which had to be seen as blinking, could be so seen if they flashed seventy-five times per minute. Blue ones could be allowed to flash only twenty times per minute, else there was danger of fusion by the dark-adapted eye of the engineer."

R. L. Gregory writes: "All eyes are primarily detectors of movement. In many forms of animal life, this is essential to survival. Man, however, though sensitive to motion, can hold his reactions under control. Indeed it now seems that it is only the eyes of the highest animals which can signal anything to the brain in the absence of movement."

There is a certain amount of retinal lag in perceiving objects and colors. Vision is not an instantaneous retinal process. When the eye scans, it does not do so in a continuous sweep but skips and hops. Stimulation at any one moment holds over to the next — and, thus, moving pictures are made possible — and visual impression remains lucid and unblurred.

But more than this occurs. In seeing any color the eye has a tendency to produce a strong response to its opposite. So pronounced is this reaction that it actually brings afterimages to view. When staring at a red area and then at a neutral surface, a sensation of green will be experienced. The afterimage of yellow will be blue. The phenomenon has great influence over color effects and gives intensity to strong contrasts and mellowness to blended color arrangements.

Recent scientific experiments indicate that afterimage effects take place in the brain rather than in the eye. This also seems true of illusions associated with brightness contrast (the fact that colors look relatively light on dark backgrounds and relatively dark on light backgrounds). With reference to afterimages, hypnotized subjects have been asked to concentrate upon color stimuli which had no literal existence. Though the subjects' eyes actually saw nothing, colors were experienced. Subjects "saw" complementary afterimages, despite the fact that their retinas had not been stimulated. Most amazing, "these were persons who, in the waking state, did not know that there is such a thing as an afterimage — let alone, that it should be expected to be complementary to the stimulus!" (Walls).

In its sensitivity to color, the human eye responds to a relatively small span of the total electromagnetic spectrum. Human vision may have had its evolution in water, for the visible spectrum is in general the transmission spectrum of water. According to Walls, "The rod spectrum is closely fitted to water, the cone spectrum a little better to air." In evolutionary terms such development is perhaps natural enough.

Though perception of color may connote spiritual, emotional, and aesthetic feelings to man, nature is less interested in beauty than in clear vision. Light and color have biological significance. Color sense aids perception. It has a functional basis and was evolved by nature not to make men happy, but to assure their better adaptation to environment. Just as nature imposes herself on man through vision, so man interprets nature as his brain directs. In short, seeing works two ways: physical stimuli from the outside world enter the eye, which then sends impulses to the brain; the brain adds its experience, judgment, and perception to what it receives, and "looks" wisely back at the world and "sees" it.

As for theories of color vision, the duplicity theory still holds weight. The rods of the eye are sensitive to brightness, while the cones react to color. It has further been postulated that the eye responds primarily to red, green, and blue wavelengths, and through combinations of them all other colors are seen.

In the retinex theory of Edwin H. Land, it is assumed that receptors in the eye operate as units to form visual records of long wavelengths and short wavelength stimuli.

In a striking experiment Land photographed a full color scene through a red filter and through a green filter to produce two separate black and white transparent prints. When red light was then projected on a screen through one black and white transparency, and when white light was also projected in register on the same screen through the other transparency, a full range of colors was seen. Land writes, "It appears, therefore, that colors in images arise not from the choice of wavelength but from the interplay of longer and shorter wavelengths over the entire scene."

In effect, this demonstration runs counter to classical color theory, which supposes that to see any given color, wavelengths of it must exist in the stimuli. However, blue wavelengths are not needed for perception to experience blue, or green wavelengths to see green. When Land used a red filter over a tungsten lamp for one image, and sodium vapor light for the other, in neither case did the light beams contain green or blue — yet the composite image was fully colored and contained blue and green.

Land's "retinexes," sensitive to brightness over hue, have much to do with color vision. The theory predicts that the eye, in seeing color in a scene, is more or less indifferent to the particular light energy or wavelengths that enter it. "We are forced to the astonishing conclusion that the rays are not in themselves color-making. Rather they are bearers of information that the eye uses to assign appropriate colors to various objects in an image."

To deal now with control of light and brightness in the environment — toward agreeable and ideal seeing conditions — here are some practical observations.

It is probably no exaggeration to say that light level is the simplest of all problems to deal with in a man-made environment. (This, of course, would exclude the technical engineering of a lighting installation.) In effect, a task is set up and light level increased until the job is visible and easily, as well as efficiently, done. Having accomplished this, however, a number of other qualifying factors arise: the surround of the task shouldn't be too dark or too bright; glare and distraction must be eliminated; some brightness should usually encompass the whole field of view; shadows should give form and depth to lighted spaces; the total "effect" must be pleasing; the appearance of the worker himself, in his setting, should be acceptable and sometimes flattering. Thus, beyond light level alone, there must be considerations as to the "quality" of the light, the color tint of the surrounding brightness, the beauty, proportion, and balance of the interior itself. (Not to forget temperature, humidity, noise level, and all the other elements that make up the indoor "climate.")

Many of the elements that demand attention are most difficult to reconcile. Even in visibility alone, what is familiar and easily recognized will not require as much light as that which is strange. Although a monotonous task, in high contrast, may require little light, the worker may be kept more alert if he is stimulated by brightness.

Many seeing tasks are tough and difficult to relieve. There is often a naïve assumption that critical seeing tasks merely need adequate light. The operation of the eye is largely muscular, and being muscular any excessive activity will tire it out — regardless of light levels or surrounding. Glare, prolonged convergence, constant shifts in accommodation, constant adjustments to extreme brightness differences, all involve wearisome muscular chores. (The retina, however, like the human brain, seems more or less immune to fatigue.)

Although light level requirements for various tasks have an extensive literature implemented by codes, specifications, and recommendations, much of this is often academic. The fact that the eye sees remarkably well over a range from 1–1000 (or more) footcandles allows for wide tolerances. Proponents of high levels may therefore speak of statistical efficiency, attempting to prove (often correctly) that the more light, the greater the accuracy.

While a person may hardly object to abundant illumination, there are nevertheless accompanying factors to consider. After all, vision is slow in dim light and needs good illumination to be fully alert. Visibility increases at a rapid rate from darkness to a 50-footcandle level. For added "efficiency" beyond this, light levels may have to be doubled and redoubled. Thus the economics of a lighting installation must be regarded, for while 50 footcandles are fairly easy to achieve, 1500 footcandles, or even 500, may cost quite a bit.

Perhaps the matter may be settled in a wholly practical way. How much would added light cost? Would the expense be offset in cash savings for added efficiency or greater freedom from accidents? Light for the sake of light has small justification. Within reasonable limits, it is very doubtful if the eye itself or the agreeable environment is involved here.

High level light may be an aid to acuity, but it may also be a handicap if the high light level involves glare or gives great brightness to wall areas. The eye cannot help itself from looking at, accommodating to, and focusing upon the brightest area in its field of view. Such response is automatic. Therefore, if walls are meaningless in the performance of a visual task, it hardly seems logical to give them the advantage.

Incidentally, H. L. Logan speaks highly of a lighting system in which 55 percent of light comes from above the horizontal line of vision and 45 percent from below. This would mean well distributed illumination, and light floors and furnishings to reflect light.

The eye is quick in adjusting itself to brightness and slow in adjusting itself to dimness. If the task is dark (as it might be), and if the surrounding is bright, the whole arrangement from the standpoint of visual efficiency and comfort may be in reverse. Some compensation, incidentally, may be achieved through color.

In any case, uniformity of stimulus is undesirable. The human organism is not adapted to unvarying stimuli. While it may seem needless to say this, many lighting codes and recommendations run contrary to very plain and obvious facts. Uniform illumination and uniform brightness in the field of vision may be ideal from an academic standpoint, but they are inconsistent with the natural properties and capabilities of human beings.

As H. L. Logan has pointed out, the human organism is in a constant state of flux. All its functions rise and ebb continually. Simple thoughts will affect respiration and pulse rate. So pronounced is this tendency for physiological and psychological experiences to fluctuate that they will take place even when the exterior world remains the same. Areas of steady brightness will appear to fade in and out. The pupil opening of the eye will actually close and dilate slightly. Steady sounds will not be heard consistently. Sensations of taste, heat, cold, and pressure will all vary and will be surprisingly independent of unvarying stimuli in the early stages of exposure. If the monotony is long continued, the ability to respond to the stimulus will deteriorate.

People require varying, cycling stimuli to remain sensitive and alert to their environments. Comfort and agreeableness are normally identified with moderate, if not radical, change, and this change concerns brightness as well as all other elements in the environment. If overstimulation may cause distress, so may severe monotony.

In simple terms, where work is performed, moderation with light or color is better than excess. If an all-white room appears sterile in the psychological sense, a black-and-white room would be objectionable in the physiological sense. Somewhere in middle ground is a better solution. The attempt to sit at the far end of a dark room and look out a window into a sunny day will result in marked discomfort. Yet if the person stirs himself to go out into the open, the same daylight may be taken in easy stride.

Both uniformity and excessive contrast are bad. An attempt by the eye to make trying adjustments may well throw it out of kilter. The road to monotony leads to visual efficiency but to emotional rejection; while the road to contrast, though it may lead to emotional acceptance, may impair good visual performance; thus, the place to meet is at the crossroads!

On good evidence, it may be said that brightness and color have two major effects. Where the task requires chief attention to the environment, high levels of general illumination and brightness in the surround will condition the human organism accordingly; the attention and interest of the room occupant will be *outward*. This would be a good principle to apply to manual tasks.

On the other hand, where the task requires concentrated visual and mental attention at fixed points (desks and work tables), softer general illumination and more subdued brightness in the surround may accomplish the best results. If critical seeing tasks are performed, supplementary localized illumination may be added. In such a setting, the attention and interest of the room occupant will be away from the environment and to the job at hand. His body and his eyes will be physiologically and optically well adjusted.

In purely casual or recreational areas, let it be added, the sky is the limit and almost anything may be done.

In the light source itself, color is all important to the truly agreeable environment. No interior, judged esthetically, could possibly be acceptably illuminated with uncorrected mercury or sodium vapor. Their cadaverous effects on human complexion would overwhelm any arguments about visibility or visual efficiency.

In nearly every study made on the chromatic quality in light as related to human appearance, warm illumination has been preferred, with ordinary incandescent light rating high. For a pleasant effect, the incandescent lamp and the deluxe, warm-white fluorescent tube would be appropriate. (Tinted bulbs go too far for general illumination and perhaps even for decorative lamps.)

After all, so-called "natural light" is an arbitrary thing. Man knows all sorts of light, from orange-pink dawn and dusk, to yellow sunlight, to white or bluish skylight. He is endowed with a special faculty (known as color constancy) to accept them all as "normal."

Illuminating engineers for the most part accept, as a standard for white light, the particular spectral characteristics of a sunny midday in June at Washington, D.C. The lighting industry has thereupon struggled to duplicate this light in artificial sources, as if it held some special magic. It is true, of course, that human beings are seldom exposed to the kind of light seen at Washington, D.C., on a noon hour in June. The orange tints of dawn and dusk are "natural light," too, as are yellow sunlight and bluish or grayish light on a cloudy day. These lighting conditions are far more average and far more prevalent. Washington June daylight isn't even necessary for color matching purposes, although it may have advantages. Color matching in industry is commonly performed under natural daylight, and such daylight varies considerably and is quite satisfactory month in and month out — and it rarely approaches the Washington June ideal.

Quite pertinent here are the very patent findings of A. A. Kruithof of Germany, that a normal appearance for object colors will require different tints in a light source, depending on the degree of illumination intensity. Kruithof's work, most important to the agreeable environment, unfortunately is little known among lighting engineers, architects, and interior designers.

In low levels of light (under 30 footcandles), object and surface colors will appear normal when the light source is slightly tinted with pink, orange, or yellow. As higher light levels are reached, a *normal* appearance for object colors will be found with cooler light that is more like sunlight or skylight at noon. Kruithof's principle is quite obvious and true. All one needs to do is to study human appearance (and colors) in dim light that is warm and dim light that is cold. The warm illumination will be "friendly" and seem wholly natural, while the cold light will seem ghastly and eerie. Even the assumption that good color discrimination demands "daylight" illumination will hold true only at high light levels, not at low ones.

So for agreeableness in illumination, it is best (and easiest) to stay warm at low levels and go cooler, if desired, at high levels. Also, some directional light should be introduced to create an interesting play of highlight and shadow. The beauty of form can be destroyed by too much "flat" lighting.

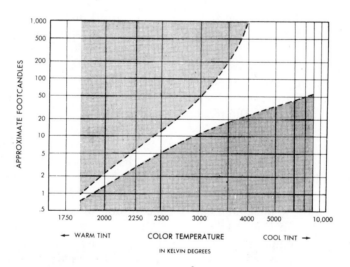

Kruithof's principle: for the environment to appear normal, use warm light at low levels of illumination, cooler light at higher.

CHAPTER FIVE

Psychological Reactions

Innumerable editorials and essays are written these days to decry the sorry state of modern architecture. Multistory office buildings file people away in cubicles like so many cardboard folders. Large scale and high-rise housing pens them up like rabbits in concrete and glass hutches. On the matter of housing, if a developer or financier allows a bit of open space for grass and shrubbery, he is extolled as a great humanitarian.

Certainly no one can complain about the ideal of letting every man have his own plot of grass under God's sky. Yet the bare facts of urbanization, the *reasons* for the dense concentrations of human beings are too often ignored. There are three population tendencies that affect architecture. First there is a widespread move to the suburbs by those fortunate souls who have climbed up the economic scale high enough to leave the caves of the cities and slums. Second, there is a trend back into the city, the reestablishment of vast housing facilities, very often in the most blighted and central areas of the metropolis.

Then third, and most curious of all, is the trend toward highrise apartments out in the country or suburbs where land lies vacant and fallow on all sides. What the essayists and many sociologists overlook is the fact that many people *like* to be jammed near their fellow men. Why does the beach at Coney Island swarm with human organisms on a summer day when adjoined stretches of sand and shore are sparsely invaded? There actually is isolation in crowds, more privacy in a box of an apartment house, where one tenant hardly ever sees and never talks to tenants next door, more seclusion than can possible be found in a suburb or out in the country, where neighborhood affairs are known to everyone.

As for architecture, the handling of population masses leaves little room for grass and bushes. Two-story units, placed at random amid playgrounds and miniparks, are out of the question. There exists in New York today a development known as Co-op City, built to house 50,000 persons. This project, on 300 acres, will have more people in it than the cities of Elmira or Poughkeepsie, each of which stretches over several square miles. All the people in suburban towns like Bronxville (7,000) or Scarsdale (18,000) could be fitted into a few buildings. How can myriads of souls be housed, if not in honeycombs! There simply isn't sufficient space to allot to nature.

The good citizens of New York who live in Co-op City are not tried, condemned, and sent there by the state; they like it and go voluntarily. Co-op City aside, it seems that people do not mind being cooped up, squeezed into elevators, lined up at checkout counters in supermarkets, infected with athlete's foot at the pool, having their progeny kicked in the stomach by the progeny of others at the community gym. This indeed is *living* for millions, and good living by their own choice and admission.

The inevitable and not-to-be-avoided crowding of people into giant ménages poses tremendous problems, among them the hazards of what is called sensory deprivation. Let this chapter now proceed to that topic in orderly fashion.

Scientists have said that, given proper food and exercise, man could survive in total darkness. This cruel sophistry that denies the purpose and significance of life itself. This writer has never heard of anyone that has been reared in total darkness. Blindness, of course, is not total darkness in the biological sense, because the body itself reacts to sunlight and absorbs sustaining radiation from it.

The big point, however, is that some scientists all too often overlook the fact that man is a psychological and psychic creature as well as a physiological one — he has a soul as well as a body.

The controlled environments that are destined to come for man have already arrived for numerous animals. While an animal, protected from predators and natural enemies, can live the proverbial life of Riley, such bliss is rarely encountered. Confinement and monotony may lead the animal to starve itself, to overeat, to refuse to procreate, to devour and destroy its kind, or any other kind.

Apes have been observed to withdraw within themselves in the manner of schizophrenics if left alone or surrounded by blank walls. Other creatures may lapse into a fatal lethargy. So it is that zoos are rapidly building better and more spacious environments with splendid results. Cubs are entering the world from parents who previously refused to breed in more austere captivity. Life spans are being increased. No doubt, important lessons are being learned for days in the future when man, too, will be an enclosed mortal who will need not only proper food and exercise, but agreeable visual sights and colors to help him maintain a pleasing and sane normality.

The physical effects of color on the human organism will induce psychological reactions. As John Ott writes, "Behind the psychological responses to color are more basic responses to specific wavelengths of radiant energy." A person is likely to feel cheerful on a sunny day and glum on a rainy one. Conversely, psychological attitudes toward color will affect bodily responses. Red may seem exciting and blue subduing. In other words, the whole of man, his body, mind, emotion, spirit, represents a coordinated unity, a microcosm, and color pervades all aspects of it. As B. J. Kouwer writes, "Color perception is not an art involving only the retina and 'consciousness' but the body as a totality."

There is just as much color within man as there is in the world beyond. While space age scientists busy themselves with interplanetary travel, other scientists in psychological realms are equally occupied with inner space. Indeed, man's knowledge of himself, his perception, mind, spirit, has been increased vastly within recent years and vies in magnitude with enlightenment on the physical aspects of the universe.

For example, with psychedelic drugs (LSD, marijuana, mescaline) colors are turned on from the inside. The brain projects them out in front, so to speak, and the spectacle may be an astounding one. Ordinary objects will take on the luster of gems. There may be spectral fountains, riotous hallucinations, and a fantastic interplay of sense responses in which colors, sounds, tastes, odors all become one animate kaleidoscope.

Although mind expanding drugs have been taken by peoples throughout the world, mostly as a part of religious ritual (peyote, mescaline, marijuana, hashish), only recently have their effects been given widespread attention. This is due, of course, to the synthetic production of such drugs as LSD. Now there has been a new vogue for psychochemicals and a new enlistment of cultists. The peyote rites of American Indians have been studied by anthropologists and other scientists. As a matter of fact, certain tribes are associated with a Native American Church in which slices of peyote take the place of the Eucharist bread. Aldous Huxley who has written brilliantly on the matter notes "that Christianity and alcohol do not and cannot mix. Christianity and mescaline seem to be more compatible."

As Huxley further remarks, "Mescaline raises all colors to a higher power and makes the percipient aware of innumerable fine shades of difference, to which, at ordinary times, he is completely blind."

According to Henrich Klüver, the most pronounced effects of mescaline (which is true also of LSD) are visual. Yet, "It is impossible to find words to describe mescal colors." They will be jewellike, luminous transparent Oriental rugs. Here is one experience described by Klüver: "Beads of different colors. Colors always changing: red to violet, green to bright gray, etc. Colors so bright that I doubt that the eyes are closed."

Sounds may create "explosions of color." However, "changes in the olfactory and gustatory fields seem to be rather infrequent." The drug apparently does not influence the sexual sphere in any specific way. "The Indian peyote-eaters maintain that it inhibits sexual desires."

Quite remarkably, Klüver tells of studies in which injections of mescaline have led to a great enlargement of visual fields in blind or nearly blind persons. "Some of the patients were enabled to read who, previous to the injection, could not; one of them went to a motion-picture show."

Reversing the procedure of psychochemical ingestion, psychedelic art and psychedelic discothèques using flashing lights, colors, fluid designs and patterns, roaring sounds, incense, attempt with fair success to blank out the real world for one of nightmarish fancy — without the taking of drugs. Let it be appreciated that, in clinical studies, flashing red lights have been found to induce seizures in epilepsy, while pulsating, stroboscopic lights are hypnotic, can produce headaches, nausea, and minor forms of a "nervous breakdown."

Even the flickering of a television set may be hazardous to some persons.

Quite on the other hand, if the sense of sight is *not* stimulated, reactions will take place anyhow. Prisoners in solitary confinement or in concentration camps, ascetic monks in the seclusion of cells, sailors who venture the oceans alone in small boats, men lost in woods or deserts, shipwrecked mortals, are often visited by colorful apparitions for no external cause. Likewise affected are persons confined to iron lungs, or otherwise immobilized by fractures and cardiac disorders. Schizophrenia is also like this. Withdrawn from humanity, hunched in a dark corner, the patient may leave his immediate world for a dream world of his own. As the psychologist R. L. Gregory states, "It seems that in the absence of sensory stimulation the brain can run wild and produce fantasies which may dominate." In the contemporary world such hallucinations may become an occupational hazard for men who sit at automated machines or who travel into empty space confined to a crowded projectile. Colors and visions from inside them may block vision of the actual environment.

In fact, sensory deprivation has introduced a new era and topic of investigation for psychiatrists and psychologists. In *The Psychology of Perception*, M. D. Vernon describes a number of fascinating clinical studies on the effects of a monotonous environment. Here is one example:

Under the direction of Hebb, at the University of MacGill, experiments were carried out to investigate the effects of keeping people for periods up to five days in a completely homogeneous and unvarying environment. In a small room they lay on a bed; they heard nothing but the monotonous buzz of machinery; they had translucent goggles over their eyes so that they could see only a blur of light; and they wore long cuffs which came down over their hands and prevented them from touching anything. Some observers were able to stay in these surroundings continuously for five days; others could not endure them for more than two days, in spite of the very high rate at which they were being paid for performing the experiment. Although at first they slept a great deal, after about a day they were unable to sleep except in snatches. They became bored and restless, and could not think in any concentrated fashion about anything. In fact, when their intelligence was tested, it was found to have deteriorated. They frequently suffered from visual and auditory hallucinations. When they emerged from their incarceration, their perceptions of their surroundings were impaired. Objects appeared blurred and unstable; straight edges, such as those of walls and floors, looked curved; distances were not clear; and sometimes the surroundings moved and swirled round them causing dizziness.

This surely speaks well for color and for reasonable exposure to other sensations in an environment. It also points out the need for variety. Blank surfaces tend to fade out if viewed continuously. Even colors may fade into neutral gray. Vision seems to degenerate unless stimulated — and so also does the mind itself drop into lethargy.

There seems to be a connection between the results of isolation and the taking of certain drugs. Woodburn Heron et al. write:

It is unlikely that the effects observed after isolation can be attributed merely to the forgetting of perceptual habits during the isolation period. They seem to resemble somewhat the effects reported after administration of certain drugs (such as mescal and lysergic acid) and after certain types of brain damage. When we consider as well the disturbances which occurred during isolation (e.g., vivid hallucinatory activity), it appears that exposing the subject to a monotonous sensory environment can cause disorganization of brain function similar to, and in some respects as great as, that produced by drugs or lesions.

To consider the astronaut, he might well be anything but rational and his senses anything but sound if he were to land on the moon after a long period of inaction. He would obviously need visual and other stimulation during his flight — and companions with whom he could check on the state of his wits.

Vernon tells further of a study conducted by H. R. Schaffer in infants under seven months of age who were hospitalized for periods of one to two weeks. The environment of the institution was monotonous and lacked variation. On being taken home, the infants continued to stare into space with blank expressions on their faces. Such behavior persisted for a few hours or for a couple of days. As Vernon summarizes:

Thus we must conclude that normal consciousness, perception, and thought, can be maintained only in a constantly changing environment. When there is no change, a state of 'sensory deprivation' occurs; the capacity of adults to concentrate deteriorates, attention fluctuates and lapses, and normal perception fades. In infants who have not developed a full understanding of their environment, the whole personality may be affected, and readjustment to a normal environment may be difficult.

Herbert Leiderman et al. have written of further hazards of isolation that center around medical care. Hospitals in particular need color as well as other sensory interests (music, TV, visitors). Leiderman and his group had volunteers willingly confine themselves up to 36 hours in a respirator in which they were able to see only a small area of ceiling. Only 5 of 17 could endure the confinement for the full 36 hours. "All reported difficulty in concentration, periodic anxiety feelings, and loss of ability to judge time. Eight of the seventeen reported some distortion of reality, ranging from pseudosomatic delusions to frank visual hallucinations. Four subjects terminated the experiment because of anxiety; two of these in panic tried to release themselves forcibly from the respirator."

What is highly pertinent here is that disturbed or ill people (not to mention sane ones, felons or others) are often expected to spend long hours and days in confined and drab quarters. Assume that a surgical operation may correct a man's illness or set a man's bones, what then if his confinement leads to other and unexpected maladies? Leiderman et al. wrote:

If normal persons can develop psychotic-like states ... how much more likely it is that sick patients, perhaps already perilously near the mental breaking point, can be tipped into psychopathological states by the stress of sensory deprivation. Delirium may be imminent for patients weakened by fever, toxicity, metabolic disturbance, organic brain disease, drug action, or severe emotional strain; sensory deprivation may tip the balance. We have accumulated clinical evidence that sensory deprivation may be one element of importance in the etiology of mental disturbance as a complication of various medical and surgical conditions.

Not only hospitals, sanitariums, but convalescent homes, nursing homes, retirement homes need to be planned to combat the frightening dangers of isolation. If old people, for example, can't stand being together with others of their kind — a situation which is usually good for them — and if they prefer solitude, such privacy must of necessity be equipped with colors, sounds, motion, or they will surely encounter neurotic disturbances.

Leiderman et al. conclude: "The therapy of sensory deprivation is actually its prevention. It may be as simple a matter as the avoidance of darkness, silence, and solitude. It may involve keeping on a night light, the provision of a radio or television set, or the presence of another person. In more complex form it would include ward organization to enhance social contact, increased attention to more stimulating hospital decor, and music, occupational, and recreational therapy."

Eyesight is surely one of life's greatest blessings. However, the Biblical parables, the dramatic legends and tales of restored sight do not invariably lead to boundless joy for those to whom vision has come again, miraculously or otherwise. R. L. Gregory writes, "Depression in people recovering sight after many years of blindness seems to be a common feature of the cases." He reports on one man of fifty-two who found difficulty in making an adjustment to sight after a successful corneal operation. What he had learned through the sense of touch apparently was contradicted when his vision was restored. "He found the world drab, and was upset by flaking paint and blemishes on things. He liked bright colors, but became depressed when the light faded. His depressions became marked, and general. He gradually gave up active living, and three years later he died."

Yet color is necessary to the total man, the psychic and spiritual one as well as the physical one.

In the design of modern environments it should be understood that color is highly important. In fact, it is ahead of form in man's unconscious regard.

To talk about people — you and I — and their feelings about color, many psychiatrists and psychologists have noted that response to form seems to arouse intellectual processes, while reactions to color are more impulsive and emotional. Small children, for example are color "dominant" more than form "dominant." In classical experiments devised by Gestalt psychologists, the ambiguous task of matching a green disk against an assortment of red disks and green triangles will readily be attempted on a basis of color by children. Adults will be hesitant and will point to the discrepancy. David Katz writes, "Color, rather than shape, is more closely related to emotion."

This primitive quality of color has been referred to by numerous investigators. Maria Rickers-Ovsiankina writes in connection with the Rorschach method: "Color experience, when it occurs, is thus a much more immediate and direct sense datum than the experience of form. Form perception is usually accompanied by a detached, objective attitude in the subject. Whereas the experience of color, being more immediate, is likely to contain personal, affectively toned notes." The rather striking observation is to

be made that the division of the spectrum into warm and cool colors holds very evident and simple meaning with reference to human personality and sense reaction. Colors seem to differ as psychic makeup differs. According to the general observations of E. R. Jaensch, with the warm color goes the primitive response of children, excitation, the extroverted human being, the predilection of the brunet complexion type. With the cool colors goes the more mature response, tranquilization, the introverted being, the predilection of the blond complexion type. Indeed, though the conclusion may be largely empirical, warmth and coolness in color are dynamic qualities, warmth signifying contact with environment, coolness signifying withdrawal into oneself. Thus what is learned from people individually may have general application in the environmental use of color.

It is unquestionably a normal condition for human beings to like color. There are precise reactions and "moods" to be associated with sunny weather, rainy weather, with a colorful world or environment and with a drab one. Yet in adults, excessive verbosity or "longing" for color may be an indication of mental confusion, for as a person grows older, interest in form quite naturally exceeds interest in color. Where there may be insistance upon balanced relationships between color and form, one probably has encountered a person who is willing to admit an emotional life but who is determined to keep it within the bounds of reason.

A person who, in general, reacts freely and agreeably to colors — any and all — is likely to have a responsive personality and to be keenly interested in if not well oriented toward the world at large. His less enthusiastic neighbor may be of solemn countenance and glum disposition. Persons having an agreeable rapport with the outer world will like color; those given to inner rapport may not.

If then, love of color is a sign of outwardly directed interests, and if indifference to color is significant of introspective tendencies, a basic though simple lesson is learned. In studies of the effects of alcohol, with the release of inhibitions in the severely introverted mortal goes also a greater response to color. Again it may be noted in empirical observation that abstract, nonobjective and surrealistic art forms, as well as modern styles of interior decor, tend to have a greater acceptance among extroverts than among introverts. The introverts are likely to prefer tradition and period styles of decor. The outwardly oriented individual may appreciate color for the sake of color; those who are inwardly oriented require a semblance of realism if art forms are to appeal to make "sense."

It may thus be generally assumed that emotionally responsive persons will react freely to color; inhibited mortals may be shocked or embarrassed by it; restricted and detached types may be unaffected.

Among the mentally ill, the significance of color has been extensively noted in case studies developed out of the Rorschach technique. There may be a reversion to childish fancies toward color. Sight of the hued test cards may cause great exuberance. Manic-depressives in particular will be pleased by color and will react with considerable (and agreeable) excitement to it.

In many forms of mental disturbance color is looked upon as an intruding and distressing element. The person may be visibly upset. He may reject the color as he would pain, close his eyes, turn from it or perhaps try to destroy it. Color shock of this nature, however, is seldom noted in manic-depressives.

Schizophrenic types are inclined to reject color, to look upon it as something which may prove "catastrophic" and break in upon their inner world. In looking at the test cards they may volunteer a few vague remarks about form but may be silent as to color.

In severe depressive states of psychotic degree, the rejection of color may be of a negative order, the person preferring a "gray" world and disdaining a colorful one. Those having the severest psychiatric defects will, as a rule, react to color but will seldom if ever see anything coherent in it.

Among epileptics, Rorschach himself noted that color response increased with the progress of disease and that it might conceivably be looked upon as a scale expressing degree of deterioration.

One of the real problems in psychiatry is to mark distinctions between psychotic reactions in which contact with reality may be lost and neurotic reaction in which contact with reality is maintained. Differences are perhaps more in degree of severity, although some clinical differences may exist.

Among emotionally disturbed persons (neurotic), it is not so much the favorable response as the unfavorable one which sets them apart from normal persons. In writing of the Rorschach test cards, Bruno Klopfer and Douglas Kelley state, "Probably the most important single sign of a neurotic reaction is color shock; . . . neurotics invariably show such shock, and only a small percentage of normals and other types of psychopathology display it."

Hysterical persons may find it difficult to organize their thoughts coherently when color is an element to be considered. The same appears true of the organically confused subject suffering from neurasthenia and exhaustion. The presence of color on the Rorschach card may elicit no more than a matter-of-fact naming of the hues, with no attempt to expose the content of thought. In anxiety states, obsessive neuroses, profound color shock may also be shown. The willingness of the hysteric to be affected by color is, perhaps, indicative of his egocentricity.

As modern civilization grows more complex, those responsible for the planning of environments will need to have a better understanding of the psychic makeup of people. While many other factors beyond color will need study, at least the specification of it can avoid mere personal fancy (of the interior designer or architect) and profit from sound research. Surely, if people are to live in controlled environments, the physical conditions (light, heat, food) can be directly and competently engineered. However, what about psychological conditions?

Carl Jung has written: "The gigantic catastrophies that threaten us are not elemental happenings of a physical or biological kind, but are psychic events. . . . Instead of being exposed to wild beasts, tumbling rocks, and inundating waters, man is exposed today to the elementary forces of his own psyche."

As for color and human responses to it, there is value in what authorities in the psychological sciences have found out about human prejudices and preferences. To quote from an article by Eric P. Mosse:

The difference between mental health and mental disease consists at last in nothing else but how this predicament is handled. The normally balanced individuum will face, brave and adapt himself to his problems, whereas mental disease is the manifestation of different depths of escape. With this fact in mind, we automatically understand why in achromatopsia of the hysterical the order in which the colors disappear, is violet, green, blue and finally red. Aside and above this experience we generally found in hysterical patients, especially in psychoneuroses with anxiety states, a predilection for green as symbolizing the mentioned escape mechanism. The emotional attack of the outside is repressed, the 'red' impulses of hatred, aggression and sex denied . . . For the same reason we will not be surprised that *red* is the color of choice of the manic and hypomanic patient giving the tumult of his emotions their 'burning' and 'bloody' expression. And we don't wonder that melancholia and depression reveal themselves through a complete 'black out.' Finally we see yellow as the color of schizophrenia. . . . This yellow is the proper and intrinsic color of the morbid mind. Whenever we observe its accumulative appearance we may be sure that we are dealing with a deep lying psychotic disturbance.

Mosse further related brown to paranoia.

Without being too symbolic, it may be said that a preference for red is to be associated with an outwardly integrated personality — or with a person who nourishes a desire to be well-adjusted to the world. Red indicates extroversion and is highly prized by persons of vital temperament. Such persons may not be too reflective and may be more ruled by impulse than by deliberation. In mental disease and psychoneuroses, red is to be associated with manic tendencies, as Mosse and others have remarked.

With yellow, however, this writer's experience would ally it more with feeble-mindedness than schizophrenia. (Schizophrenics generally prefer blue.) It is likely to be preferred by persons having an intellectual bent. In other words, yellow may be looked upon as an intellectual color, associated both with great intelligence and mental deficiency. Vincent Van Gogh's attraction to the hue is notable in many of his paintings, particularly in those executed in the latter years of his life. The abstract painter Kandinsky wrote with some fervor: "Yellow is the typically earthly color. It can never have profound meaning. An intermixture of blue makes it a sickly color. It may be paralleled in human nature with madness, not with melancholy or hypochondriacal mania, but rather with violent, raving lunacy."

Green may, with a generous empirical viewpoint, be associated with Freud's oral character. At least, it is often the choice of persons who are superficially intelligent, social, who are given to voluble habits of speech, and who often have an intense appetite for food. To the psychoneurotic and psychotic, green is a great favorite. Probably it suggests escape from anxiety, sanctuary in the untroubled greenness of nature. Under stress those who prefer green will not as a rule crave seclusion; on the contrary they may seek out and need companionship.

Narcissism is, in a surprisingly high percentage of cases, revealed by a preference for blue-green. Where an average mortal will like either green or blue, the choice of blue-green may indicate fastidiousness, sensitiveness, and discrimination. The need of such persons is more to be loved than to love; because of a pronounced self-love and self-sufficiency, the writer has been told that they are often difficult patients for the psychiatrist.

Blue is the color to be associated with schizophrenia. A majority of inwardly-integrated personalities will favor the color, for it is to be allied with a conscious control of emotions. Here is the color of circumspection. Under stress persons who like blue may tend to make a tragic flight from environment.

With brown the anal character of Freud is fairly well symbolized: conscientiousness, parsimony, obstinacy. Brown, of course, is to be associated with human excrement.

There are many other aspects to color preferences. Convivial persons may be attracted to orange; artistic persons may prefer purple. A well disciplined red personality may expose his imposed training by a preference for maroon. In what the psychiatrist terms the liberation of repressed effects, a meek, shy soul may take to brilliant hues with "fire in his eye." The aggressive mortal to whom life has been a tough and harsh struggle may be drawn to the tint of pink. To him pink may be a bright symbol of an unconscious wish for gentility.

While many of the above observations concern the reactions of individual persons — and people are quite unalike — it is possible to organize a knowledgeable approach to color that avoids hunch or personal fancy for a more objective attention to human needs.

For example, it is a fallacious tradition (shared by interior designers) to recommend cool colors for excitable persons and warm colors for phlegmatic ones. In small children, a pacific environment and pacific attitude may serve only to increase tension and prod irritability. Here bright color may relieve nervousness by creating an outward stimulus to balance an inner and wholly natural fervor. Conversely, in melancholy humans an attempt to "cheer up" a mood of dejection (through color or anything else) may serve merely to aggravate the misery and drive it even deeper. For most of us, at least, an extroverted temperament may be content in a bright and colorful environment, while an introverted temperament may find greatest peace in a more sedate and conservative setting.

The second part of this book sets forth practical color specifications for environments of several kinds. To anticipate how, in some instances, sound principles may be followed, here are two simple conclusions.

First, there is in color and light what might be called a centrifugal action — away from the organism, to its environment. With high levels of illumination, warm and luminous colors in the surroundings (yellow, peach, pink), the body tends to direct its attention outward. There is increased activation in general, alertness, outward orientation. Such an environment is conducive to muscular effort, action, and cheerful spirit. It is a good setting for factories, schools, homes where manual tasks are performed or where sports are engaged in.

Second, on the other hand, color and light may have a centripetal action — away from the environment and toward the organism. With softer surroundings, cooler hues (gray, blue, green, turquoise) and lower brightness, there is less distraction and a person is better able to concentrate on difficult visual and mental tasks. Good inward orientation is furthered. Here is an appropriate setting for sedentary occupations requiring severe use of the eyes or brain — offices, study rooms, fine assembly in industry.

Much of interior architecture and most of interior design has been an art rather than a science. Schools and colleges have encouraged initiative and originality. Conformance to the past has often been looked upon as a form of indolence and evil. There is nothing wrong in this attitude. Surely man is not to keep repeating himself. However, to be different is not necessarily to be better. An architect who designs a school according to idea A will probably try another idea, B, for a second school, and idea C for a third. Despite the passage of time, school C will not, for this reason, be superior to school A, except that bad mistakes may be rectified. Progress through the years is not always up; sometimes it falters and goes down.

With the average interior designer, there seems to be an eternal quest for the unique and startling. Personality and individuality must be encouraged. As a consequence the needs of a particular problem may be overshadowed by the egotism of the designer. In a recent hospital project a designer, in a press release, disdained as "rubbish" certain acknowledged principles having to do with brightness relationships for comfortable vision and restrained brilliance of hue for emotional ease. Many walls had to be repainted and many corrections made. Vermilion may be a charming and delightful color on casual view, but expose a distraught patient to it and nerves may be upset — like scratching on glass. Or let a fashionable yellow-green cast its reflections on a jaundiced mortal and he may think himself far closer to the grave.

While architecture itself is closely allied to engineering, architectural and interior *design* all too often allow impulse and taste to dominate reason. Among interior designers there is much envy and little agreement as to what is good and what is bad. This situation will no doubt always prevail. It is a fair situation where the designer may be doing a home, a shop, a restaurant, a theater. Here great individuality may well result in great commercial success.

Yet offices, schools, hospitals, mass housing are another matter. People, young and old, well and ill, are not being entertained. Most are trying to perform useful work, learn something, be cured of ailments, be spared isolation and dejection. It hardly seems proper to guess what might be best for them. What they require in an environment can be analyzed and studied and not merely surmised.

The architect, fortunately, is now calling upon the services of sociologists and psychiatrists to aid him in understanding such things as the space requirements of human beings. Most interior designers, however, have yet to request such counsel. The functionally right environment of the future will demand adequate biological lighting, temperature and noise control, efficient traffic regulation and space relationships, colors and color effects that counteract monotony and are meaningful beyond beauty alone. There will be a meeting of minds, knowledge and experience — perhaps under the overall supervision and guidance of an outstanding man.

In the realm of light and color, the chapters that now follow are meant to offer factual and practical guidance, to which the architect and interior designer can add as much of their own personality as they wish. The important point in the opinion of this writer is that a very thorough and scholarly attempt has been made to bring together for review a wealth of relevant facts, data and observations. These the reader can absorb in whole or part, accept or reject as he sees fit. But he will have, it is hoped, a fairly broad base of reference, thoughts that may not have occurred to him, points of view that may have small or large value in his professional endeavors.

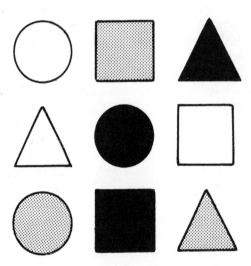

The experiment of David Katz: should one sort by color or shape?

CHAPTER SIX

Biological Lighting

Let the direction of this book now shift toward practical applications of color and lighting — supported by the research and evidence so far presented. In his professional activities, this writer has endeavored to be student, scholar, and practitioner of color relationships all in one. He has been less concerned with the sciences of physics or chemistry than with physiology, psychology, and human reactions in general. He has worked with color and people for several decades, doing his best to adapt the pure, scientific inquiries of others to everyday problems and conditions.

To begin with the all-important matter of lighting, if man-made environments may keep people out of nature and away from the sun — if not for all their lives but for long periods of it — then man-made light sources will have to take nature's place and provide the radiant energy needed to sustain life. Efforts in this direction have already made progress in the lighting industry.

Visible light and the adjacent infrared and ultraviolet regions of it are essential to the growth and health of plants, insects, fish, birds, animals, and men. There is balance, a continuous life-supporting spectrum, the different parts of which have different effects. What these effects are have been discussed in previous chapters, and more will be submitted now.

It must be admitted, however, that with proper diet and exercise, man can exist fairly well without light. Yet where he is deprived of light, he survives none too well. His sexual maturity is affected, his metabolism upset, and he is destined for an earlier death.

Where he may be blind but exposed to light, he will fare better. His flesh will absorb radiation from the sun to form vitamin D. Radiation may also penetrate his eye sockets and skull and stimulate the functioning of his glands. His entire sympathetic nervous system will be agreeably prodded.

However, rarely have men been known to spend a lifetime in total darkness, blind or not. It is conceivable that the individual man, and the race of man, would perish.

To consider more normal situations, man needs light in order to see and in order that his physical well being will be safeguarded. He doesn't need a great deal of light in either case. People who dwell in the tropics do not live longer than people in colder and less sunny latitudes. Richard J. Wurtman has written, "The 'tone' of at least a portion of the sympathetic nervous system responds to environmental lighting, mediated via the retina." In fact, studies are now being undertaken to verify the theory and belief that the retina contains nerve endings not primarily related to vision, their purpose being to stimulate the pineal gland (as well as other glands) and in turn to regulate and release substances such as hormones and enzymes into the bloodstream. The entire body of man is thus healthfully animated.

In the controlled environment, what qualities of light and radiant energy should be utilized for favorable biological responses in human beings? To answer the question first in a negative sense, there is risk in *not* exposing man to certain bands of wavelengths. John Ott in experiments with mice has clearly shown that prolonged and restricted exposure to pink light can cause death. Here Ott attributes the lethal effect not so much to red itself but to *lack* of exposure to green, blue, and ultraviolet. The light, being out of balance, so to speak, throws the bodily functions of the animal out of kilter and the animal dies.

Most artificial environments today expose people to unbalanced light sources. Incandescent light is almost completely lacking in ultraviolet wavelengths. The glass tubes of most fluorescent lighting fixtures absorb and screen out ultraviolet. Some mercury sources, rich in ultraviolet, lack red and infrared frequencies. (Clear mercury lighting, however, is objectionable because of the distortion of colors in an environment and the ugly appearance of human complexion.)

Most commonly employed artificial light sources today afford fair if not ideal frequencies throughout the *visible* spectrum, red, orange, yellow, green, blue. This is the natural consequence of human demand for white light that will assure good visibility and good appearance for environmental colors. Infrared, which may be weak in fluorescent sources, will probably exist in the energy emitted by incandescent lamps, steam radiators, or any warm or hot surfaces in an interior. Even air conditioning systems will not cancel radiant heat rays — but only their warming action on air and atmosphere.

So the current need in artificial light sources for the most part settles down to ultraviolet and how much of it should be given to man for a salubrious biological result. Simply, most "white" light today automatically covers most of the visible spectrum range. (People would hardly accept light that wasn't white and which didn't therefore reveal the world in its true colors by having wavelengths of red, yellow, green, blue in its composition.) But most "white" light is deficient in ultraviolet. Hence, if ultraviolet energy is to be added for a desirable biological balance, consideration must be given to this particular region of the electromagnetic spectrum.

The ultraviolet radiation that lies next to visible violet can be conveniently classified as long wave or short wave. Long wave ultraviolet (adjacent to visible violet) will produce fluorescence in many substances. It is responsible for the fluorescent lamp or tube, activating phosphors which become highly luminous. Other waves cause suntan. As the waves grow still shorter, erythema of the skin is caused. Here cholesterol is activated in the body and vitamin D generated. Where quartz is substituted for glass (which absorbs ultraviolet), energy is produced which will kill germs, sterilize liquids and foods, generate ozone, and perform other marvels.

While ultraviolet has many uses in industry because of its photochemical action, the interest in this chapter is directed toward human environments. It should be understood that undue exposure to ultraviolet can cause much harm to the body and be hazardous to the eyes. At the same time, its beneficial effects, such as in the formation of vitamin D, are highly efficacious. Balance is forever necessary. (Some types of bacteria, for example, are essential to life on earth and should not be destroyed.)

To get down to cases, here are some practical notes regarding the introduction of ultraviolet radiation in controlled environments.

There are bactericidal lamps which may be used to destroy airborne germs. These can be installed in room interiors or in air ducts. In reflectors, aluminum is most efficient. Such sources should perhaps be shielded so that the energy does not directly shine on human flesh or into human eyes. Applications can be made to hospital operating rooms, recovery rooms, private rooms and wards, corridors, kitchens. In school classrooms and general offices, contamination through airborne microorganisms can be controlled. In high humidity areas, bakeries, breweries, and the like, bactericidal lamps will reduce mold and cross infections. (They can also be used to sterilize liquids, water, pharmaceuticals, foods.)

Friedrich Ellinger offers this report on a naval training center in his book, *Medical Radiation Biology:* "A study of the influence of air sterilization of mass-living quarters extended over a number of years gave the following results: Ultraviolet radiation of the floors and upper air in barracks housing recruits resulted in a 19.2% overall reduction in total respiratory disease. Streptococcus disease rates were at a very high level and a 24% reduction was obtained. The reduction was fairly consistent throughout the season." However, the investigators did not feel justified in extending the application, despite encouraging results.

Perhaps the lighting problem from the biological standpoint should not be handled separately from two positions — visible light for seeing, and ultraviolet radiation for vitamin D formation and air sterilization. Rather, the plan should be all-embracing. And moderate amounts of ultraviolet should undoubtedly be part of the general interior lighting scheme — and maybe in one type of lighting unit only.

Such a unit is now on the market in a fluorescent source known as Vita-Lite, a "general purpose bulb that includes both visible and ultraviolet spectrum." (The manufacturer is the Duro-Test Corporation of North Bergen, New Jersey.)

Without referring specifically to Vita-Lite, the benefits of a balanced light source — which includes some ultraviolet energy — can be duly recommended and will no doubt be further developed and perfected and made an integral part of the controlled environment of the future.

Man evidently needs a reasonable amount of ultraviolet radiation — on his body and into his eye — to lead a healthful life. What happens? To quote again from Ellinger:

Irradiation of human subjects with erythema producing doses of ultraviolet resulted in an improvement of work output. In studies on the bicycle-ergometer, it has been shown that under these laboratory conditions, the work output could be increased up to 60%. Analysis of this phenomenon revealed that the increased output is due to decreased fatigability and increased efficiency. Cardiovascular responses served as an indicator. In the irradiated subjects the pulse rate returned more rapidly to normal values after physical exercise. Irradiation of subjects with filtered ultraviolet light sources proved that the increase in work output is caused by the total ultraviolet content and is dependent only on the production of erythema irrespective of whether produced by the long or short wave type.

There is much to ponder over in this statement. Ultraviolet opens up the pores of the skin, stimulates circulation, produces vitamin D, prevents rickets, increases protein metabolism, causes a drop in blood pressure, affects and stimulates the glands, lessens fatigue, and otherwise gives man quite a physiological and even psychological boost. But its specification and prescription demands caution, care, and the counsel of an experienced and scientifically trained authority in the radiobiological field.

Finally, here is the statement of two Russian scientists, N. M. Lazarev and M. V. Sokolov, at a meeting in 1967 of the International Congress on Illumination at Washington, D. C.:

If the human skin is not exposed to solar radiation (direct or scattered) for long periods of time, disturbances will occur in the physiological equilibrium of the human system. The result will be functional disorders of the nervous system and a vitamin-D deficiency, a weakening of the body's defenses, and an aggravation of chronic diseases. Sunlight deficiency is observed more particularly in persons living in the polar regions and in those working underground or in windowless industrial buildings.

The simplest and at the same time the most effective measure for the prevention of this deficiency is the irradiation of human beings by means of ultraviolet lamps. Such irradiation is conducted either in special rooms called photaria or directly in locations where persons are regularly present — in workshops, schools, hospitals, etc. As a rule, the daily dosage of ultraviolet does not exceed half of the average dose which produces a just perceptible reddening of an untanned human skin. It is preferable to use fluorescent lamps which use phosphor and have a maximum emission of 315 nm. The beneficial effect of ultraviolet irradiation has been confirmed by many years of experience.

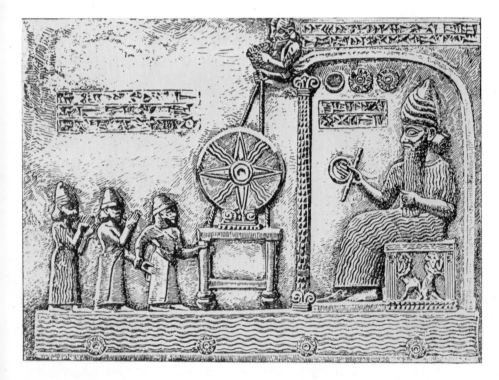

A Sun worship, drawn from an ancient relief sculpture.

CHAPTER SEVEN

Good Vision Lighting

The subject of this chapter has been featured, stressed, and belabored by illuminating engineers over many years. Literature on the matter is profuse and quite out of proportion to the size of the problem itself. Through sheer persistence and verbosity on the part of the lighting industry, many architects, interior designers, and building owners have been prevailed upon to raise light levels to rather astonishing and bewildering heights. And quite often people exposed to this light have tinkered with it, screened it, and cut it down to reasonable intensity.

How much light is necessary for clear and comfortable seeing? Specious arguments have often been presented to the effect that a rising rate of eye and vision deficiencies is to be traced to inadequate light. Much of this is sophistry. Kerosene lamps, gaslight, and electricity itself did not become sources of illumination until the end of the nineteenth century. Before that, and for many, many centuries, men relied on tallow and oil lamps, candles, fire, and they saw quite well indeed, to judge from their surviving works. If man's eyesight is breaking down these days (which is questionable), this would not be due to lack of light but to his occupation with more difficult and trying eye tasks.

Chapter 4 has discussed human vision and has set forth a number of principles that concern lighting and visual efficiency and comfort. The purpose now is to offer further notes on lighting as they relate to good vision and to extend practical counsel in the creation of man-made environments.

If man needs high levels of light in the future, it will be more for biological reasons than for visual ones. Many a scribe and scholar in the dim past has done remarkably fine work under dim candlelight — the light of one candle one foot from his task. Who can argue that he would have done far better with 500 or 1000 footcandles!

According to acceptable history in the lighting industry, about 70 years ago Herman Cohn of Germany came to the conclusion that approximately 1 footcandle was the satisfactory minimum for reading 8-point type in black on white. Some fifty or more years ago in 1917, M. Luckiesh, a prominent American authority, gave 3-6 footcandles as the optimum in libraries. A. P. Trotter, in 1921, specified a required 3-4 footcandles for library tables. In 1923, J. W. T. Walsh wrote, "For reading and writing, it is now generally agreed than an illumination of about three footcandles is the most comfortable." And in 1924, the so-called Geneva Code of the International Congress on Illumination recommended 5 footcandles as the minimum for school library tables.

Yet by 1941, lighting engineers were claiming that "250 footcandles for reading appears to be below the optimum for easiest reading." Still later, up to today, levels as high as 500 footcandles have become quite ordinary.

Now, however, this matter has come full circle. Dr. H. R. Blackwell, in studies sponsored by the Illuminating Engineering Society, has reported that the illumination necessary to give 8-point type a "suprathreshold visibility of 15, and to afford a visual capacity of five assimilations per second with the maximum accuracy (99 percent) is, according to the fount, 1.13 or 1.87 footcandles." So it is that Blackwell ends up where earlier investigations started.

Perhaps high light levels accompany progress in general. They definitely make seeing easier, quicker, and more efficient. But beyond a level of about 100 or 150 footcandles, they really aren't necessary. In fact, they well may cause trouble. If the light sources are not well screened, if there is excessive brilliance overhead, white or off-white glare from walls, specular reflections, man in his environment may suffer. Two experts in the field of vision, C. E. Ferree and Gertrude Rand, wrote as follows a number of years ago:

The presence of a bright source of light or other surface of high brilliancy in the field of view produces a blinding effect through a phenomenon known as irradiation; that is, the source seems to be surrounded by a broad and intense halo of light, the intensity of which falls off as the source is receded from. This serves to confuse and blur seeing in direct relation to the intensity of the source and in inverse relation to its distance from the line of sight and the brightness of the remainder of the field of vision. Two causes of this phenomenon may be noted: the scattering of light by the refracting media of the eye which serves to throw an overlay of unfocused light on the image of the working surface; and an induction or spreading of the excitation on the retina produces a similar overlay in sensation.

The presence of high brilliancies in the field of view produces disturbances in the control of the mechanism of the adjustment of the eye which rapidly lead to the fatiguing of the muscles of adjustment, and the loss of power to sustain the precision of adjustment needed for clear seeing . . .

Brilliancies, if too high, may cause an actual damage to the retina itself. These may take the form of congestions and inflammations, scotoma, detachments, etc.

In conclusion, light sources, of high or low intensity, should be placed out of sight and properly baffled with louvers or lenses. Walls should not be white in an environment where critical eye tasks are performed. If the work task requires a great deal of light, a localized source may be introduced — but never in a dark room. Miniature, high-intensity lamps, popular these days, can raise havoc with vision if they are used in an otherwise dim surround.

As for general light levels, the Illuminating Engineering Society publishes guides to recommended practice. For offices, levels from 20 footcandles for corridors, to 30 for casual tasks, to 70 for reading and transcribing, to 100 for regular office work, to 150 for accounting, to 200 for designing and drafting, are reasonable and acceptable. The same levels are more or less also proper for schools. Recommended reflectances for surfaces should range from about 20% for floors to 25-40% for furniture, to 40-60% for walls, to 80-90% for ceilings — and again these are reasonable and acceptable. (Special end wall treatments could safely be in the 25-40% reflectance range.)

In hospitals, light levels may range from 5-10 footcandles for recovery rooms, patients' rooms and wards, to 1,000, 2,000 or 2,500 footcandles (localized) for operating rooms. Laboratory areas, where visual work tasks are performed, should have from 50–100 footcandles.

Light should neither be too directional (like a beam of sunlight) nor too diffuse (like a cloud). In one instance severe highlights and shadows may be created, and in the other a sense and awareness of three dimensional forms may be lost or confused. While indirect lighting is soft and appealing in many applications, it is quite inefficient in output. Direct light, on the other hand, while efficient in output, may create glare by shining too starkly on tasks and leaving a dim overhead. A direct-indirect, or semi-direct system is perhaps best of all. Some light is directed upward and some downward for a fairly uniform spread of brightness. Where troffer or other types of lighting covers an entire ceiling, clear prism lenses, or egg crates, or baffles of low diffuse reflectance are requisite for adequate comfort.

In work spaces (offices, schools, industrial plants) dark ceilings are objectionable, despite their esthetic appeal. Yet in decorative use (homes, exclusive shops, restaurants, bars, recreation areas) the dark ceiling is admissible and may be quite handsome.

Regarding visibility under different light sources, Luckiesh points out that yellow is in the region of maximum selectivity, the brightest portion of the spectrum. It is without aberration (that is, the eye normally focuses it perfectly), and it is psychologically pleasing. By experiment, Luckiesh also demonstrated that by filtering out blue and violet radiation in a mercury light (also, in a tungsten lamp), visual acuity remained practically constant, despite the reduced amount of light absorbed by the filter. This would mean that, as far as visual acuity is concerned, yellow has definite advantages. Sodium light, for example, is highly efficient, although its distortion of colors makes it impossible for use under many circumstances.

Ferree and Rand placed yellow illumination at the top of the list, orange-yellow second, followed by yellow-green and green. Deep red, blue, and violet were least desirable. Blue, in fact, is very difficult for the eye to focus and will cause objects to appear blurred and surrounded by halos.

Under extreme dark adaptation, however, the eye seems to have best acuity under red light. Red illumination has been widely used for instrument panels in airplanes, for control rooms on ships and submarines. It has little influence on the dark-adapted eye and is not, in fact, seen on the outer boundaries of the retina, where the cones are lacking. It is therefore suitable as a blackout illuminant and will fail to stimulate the eye except when its rays strike near the fovea.

Finally, here are a few comments regarding color and vision. First, what colors are most easily seen? Yellow is the point of highest visibility in the spectrum, the region where there is greatest brightness and where acuity is sharp. Next in order would be orange, red, yellow-green. In air-sea rescue, red-orange is the color used because of greater contrast against water and whitecaps.

Yet there may be a difference between visibility and recognition. White, for example, holds little visual interest perhaps because of its lack of "chromaticity" and because it does not have the dynamic qualities of the spectral hues. In studies devoted to light signals, red is first in recognition and the easiest color to identify. Next is green, then yellow, then white. Blue and violet are of little consequence here. In average experience, white is a difficult color either to remember or to find. It is weak in compulsion, and although it may be seen at greater distances, the eye finds difficulty in seizing upon it.

In attention, red-orange perhaps ranks first, followed by red, yellow, and certain luminous tones of green and pink. There is little doubt about the merits of red-orange in stimulating vision. It is the color of greatest vividness and impact and is quite impossible to disregard — it will draw the eye despite everything.

Size is a function of brightness. Yellow will be seen as the largest, then white, red, green, blue, black. Pastels will likewise be larger than shades. The reason for this is quite simple. Brightness, when it strikes the nerves on the retina of the eye, tends to spread out like a drop of water on blotting paper. Thus it will form a larger image than will anything dark.

In dimension, near to far, the warm colors will advance, while the cool colors will retire. Here again optic laws are involved. Being only slightly refracted by the lens of the eye, red will focus at a point behind the retina. To see it clearly, the lens will grow more convex, thus pulling the color forward, making its image larger. Blue will be more sharply refracted and will cause the lens of the eye to flatten out. This will push the image of blue back and decrease its size.

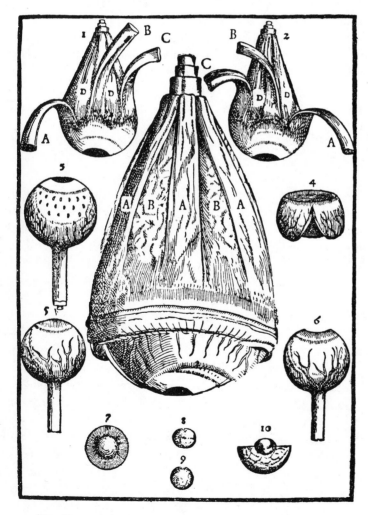

Woodcuts of the human eye, from a 16-century text.

CHAPTER EIGHT

Lighting for Appearance

It would seem from the last two chapters that lighting in the controlled environment should, for biological reasons, emit a measure of long and short wave ultraviolet, and that for clear visibility intensity should be at a level of 50, 100, or more footcandles, depending on work task. Lighting engineers, however, all too often forget or disregard the factor of appearance. What is the spectral quality of the light? How do things appear under it? How do *people* look? Regarding this latter question, G. B. Buck and H. C. Froehlich have written, "There is one surface, the average human complexion, which presents itself under nearly every lighting installation and which consciously or unconsciously often becomes the criterion by which the job is evaluated." In one personal experience of this writer (Birren) women employed to work in an industrial area illuminated by clear mercury reported severe "eyestrain" and distress. While light level was perfectly ample, the complaint was easily traced to the fact that the complexions of the women turned greenish and their lips black — and this was hardly tolerable in a situation where men were also present.

One of the most naive assumptions regarding illumination, frequently shared by lighting engineers, architects, building owners, and laymen, is that it ought to be as close as possible to natural daylight. If the room or area demands accurate color discrimination, imitation natural daylight may be necessary. But let it be fully appreciated that such light sources are far from flattering to human complexion, which will turn sallow and grayish under their influence. Indeed, the proverbial use of cosmetics (before the advent of green and blue eye shadow and white lipstick) was to daub pink powder on the skin and to apply red rouge to the cheeks and lips — to accent what most women considered to be nature's intention. Researchers have also found that human memory of true complexion color is substantially on the pinkish side. That's why artists forever accentuate rich ruby bloom. C. L. Sanders further determined that people actually prefer complexion tints that are ruddier than the actual tone of their own flesh.

In another experience of this writer, general lighting in a large retail store having no partitions had to be adjusted, both in the women's fashion department and in furniture. While cool white fluorescent tubes gave fairly accurate color values to dresses, the female customer in seeing herself in a mirror looked pallid. And because of this the dress looked "awful" and was likely to be rejected. Store management found a better policy in using deluxe warm white lamps in the dress department in order to flatter the buyer, despite the color distortion of the clothing donned by the customer. In furniture the fluorescent lamps were removed entirely, the area being illuminated by floor and table lamps, plus a number of choicely located reflectors and urns holding incandescent bulbs — just like at home.

After all, it is invalid to conclude that daylight types of light sources assure true color rendition. They will hold this merit only when light intensity is at a high level. In Chapter 4 reference was made to the work of A. A. Kruithof who very aptly and correctly noted that the objects and surfaces of the world will have a "normal color appearance" under *warm* light at low levels of intensities and *cool* light under high levels. In nature dim light, such as at sunrise and sunset, is usually warm and golden in hue. So is firelight. As daylight reaches higher levels, it shifts in tint from pink, to orange, to yellow, and finally into white or even blue, as from a north sky in summer. Throughout these shifts in hue, as the light level rises, the colors of objects continue to look normal. That is, no person will find the changing scene to be at all unnatural. In effect, white or daylight illumination *at low levels* will cast an eerie and altogether weird pallor over the world — while warm light at the same low levels will seem wholly proper.

Thus, for the sake of good appearance, warm light at low levels and cooler or whiter light at high levels should be regarded in the controlled environment. Some lamp manufacturers, such as General Electric, are aware of this. Incandescent bulbs and warm white fluorescent tubes are noted as having "greater preference at lower levels," while cool white, daylight, and color-corrected mercury lamps have "greater preference at higher levels."

Candlelight, real or simulated, is notable for the "cozy," friendly and intimate atmosphere. Cool daylight, at high levels, is well recommended for work tasks and for the sale of merchandise. A cocktail lounge would suggest live ghouls and dead ghosts, if illuminated by dim blue or violet light, whereas a school classroom or office under brilliant red or pink light would be visually and psychologically objectionable — just as there are objections to sodium vapor light (yellowish) or clear mercury (greenish), whenever and wherever human complexion and appearance are judged. Various effects of different tints in light sources and the influences of colored backgrounds on human complexion are shown in Color Plate I.

The makers of illuminating tubes and lamps have, on occasion, published charts describing and illustrating the changes that take place when "white" light sources of different tint are caused to shine on surfaces of different color. Such data for the most part are academic and misleading. First of all, where light booths or boxes are set up to show, *simultaneously*, the different effects of different light sources, the very magic of human vision is denied. In a phenomenon known as color constancy, the world of color tends to maintain a *normal* appearance under widely varying conditions of light intensity and hue. A white surface does not look pink at dawn, yellow under sunlight, or blue under reflected sky light — unless critical examination is insisted upon or unless other tinted illuminants are introduced at the same time. Sitting in an office under incandescent light, another office across a street or court illuminated by fluorescent light will appear bluish. Or in the reverse situation, the incandescent-lit office will look yellowish to anyone sitting in a fluorescent-lit room. The eye and the brain adjust themselves quite well to changes in light intensity and hue, and they do remarkably well in holding the world to a "normal" appearance at all times.

As charts and tables in the lighting industry often describe, daylight types of illumination (bluish) will naturally enhance the purity or charm of blue and green colors. Incandescent light or warm white fluorescent will, in a similar way, add richness to red, orange, and yellow. Yet this is all of minor concern in the phenomenon of color constancy. What so often is important is simply this: how do people look? Would anyone for the sake of a blue wall, carpet, or tablecloth, illuminate a room with blue tinted light and at the same time make people look nauseated!

Bear in mind that people will have a subjective as well as objective attitude toward color and tinted light. Most persons regard blue and green as being cool and restful, *out there in the world*. But blue or green flesh tones are for cadavers, not live people.

For their vanity, people like warm illumination. Stage lighting is essentially orange in quality, so is the lighting commonly found in restaurants, bars, hotel rooms, hospital rooms, and homes.

In the early days of fluorescent light, most of which was bluish, it went into bathrooms and kitchens and then went out. Now the lighting industry has developed "complexion" and "candlelight" tints, and all is well again.

Yet most people go to work, engage in useful tasks, and do not merely sit about looking into mirrors or into each other's eyes. Sodium vapor lighting is quite acceptable for highways. For many years high bay industrial areas have used clear mercury. Here the workingman (or woman) is not concerned over personal appearance. The lighting industry, however, and to good cause, continues to try to achieve more agreeable lighting in its highly efficient high intensity lamps. On the market today are excellent mercury sources, plus a new Lucalox (General Electric) lamp, which is particularly efficient but which, unlike mercury, has a pleasing golden yellow tint. While this particular lamp may not lead to true color fidelity, it is a good one to consider for places where large masses of people are assembled — and who look at each other. This would include gymnasiums, natatoriums, sports arenas, playgrounds, parking lots. Flesh under it looks yellowish, but not ashen, grayish, or greenish.

In lighting there is, as mentioned, an objective attitude toward color — how colors and surfaces look in the world beyond — and a subjective attitude — how they look on human flesh. Often in working environments the objective view is maintained. In a study by W. G. Pracejus for the General Electric Company, two office type rooms, about 14 x 17 feet, were set up, one in a warm color effect and one in a cool. Light level was set at about 100 footcandles, but different sources were employed. The rooms were then occupied for periods of about 90 minutes by office personnel who undertook actual work. Results for short-term or long term occupancy showed little difference.

Seven test light sources were used; fluorescent cool white, deluxe cool white, white, and warm white; two types of mercury light; and one type of sodium discharge. Personal reactions to the seven kinds of illuminants were then recorded for 1,543 observations. Greatest preference was shown for the fluorescent cool white. Of the other sources there was little difference among deluxe cool white, white, warm white, and the color-corrected mercury. Only the sodium vapor discharge lamp ranked low.

One could assume from this that cool types of fluorescent light sources are quite satisfactory for *working environments* (with perhaps some ultraviolet included for good health).

Flattery indexes have recently been discussed in the lighting field.

Deane B. Judd has considered the appearance of such things as human complexion, butter, foliage, green grass. When memory is called upon, average persons will think of flesh as being redder than it usually is, butter as being yellower, and grass as being bluer (less yellowish) than in nature. While preference attitudes toward such things as paints, textiles, furniture, floor coverings have wide tolerance limits, greater discrimination will be shown toward foods. Here meat, dairy goods, vegetables, fruits, bakery products must be *just so* or they will be rejected. Green meat, orange butter, gray fruit, purple bread would discourage any normal appetite.

Color Plate I offers an interesting graphic picture of the effect of different light sources on human complexion—as well as the influence of different background colors under the same light source. In large-scale architectural projects (offices, schools, hospitals) it is desirable to use more than one type of illuminant in the various areas: low-level warm light in rest areas; higher-level warm light for food service; cooler and still higher light for working areas. A mixture of incandescent spots with fluorescent overhead lighting also offers good possibilities: It allows for highlights and shadows, subtle shifts in color tint, and reduction of flatness and monotony.

CHAPTER NINE

Psychic Lighting

Lighting for emotional, psychological, and psychic effects has suddenly become a new art form. For the most part, man has been an observer of environments created by others; now he would participate in environments and form them himself. He could, for example, sit at a console in an all-white room and project patterns, colors, movement at will to satisfy his innate desires. Of if he were a great artist, he could stir the feelings of others with visions that were akin to the emotional effects of sounds and music.

The fact that colors have physiological and emotional effects has been fairly well covered in the first chapters of this book. Man responds to his environment and at times may be helpless within it. Perhaps the most distressing of all experiences is to be in no environment at all, or in a bleak environment of unrelieved monotony. Next would be the environment of a riotous nightmare from which there was no escape.

The psychic environment of today, chiefly noted for light, color, and sound, has been inspired by the recent and widespread indulgence in hallucinogenic drugs, marijuana, peyote, mescalin, LSD, psilocybin, and other psychochemicals. One of the first manifestations of them is a wondrous blaze of color. As described by Weston La Barre, "Time perception is altered and a curious double existence occurs. One part of the mind remains critical and well oriented, but when the eyes are closed and opened, elaborately beautiful designs are seen — fields of brilliantly colored jewels, vast and showly changing geometrical constructions."

Whether or not the taking of hallucinogens will become a national habit (or menace), one thing is quite certain: the experience of taking "acid" or "pot" has already become a part of the American and world scene. With the advent of psychedelic art, the discothèque, a good part of man's environment may well be due for revolutionary change. And when the change comes, light will be a vital part of it.

What is most significant is that the *simulation* of mind expanded states can be induced; one does not have to take LSD. Turn up the lights, the colors, the sounds, and people can be emotionally transported. Maybe the basic impetus to the psychedelic way centers around the universal conviction that outer life is a hopeless and futile mess, so let's get away from it and into another world of inner splendor.

Psychedelic experience is to be created by the use of lights, colors, motion pictures, slides, projectors, strobes, oscilloscopes, stereo tapes, mechanically produced sounds, plus the thump of a beating heart. Put them all together and the excitement and distraction may be so compelling as to lift a person completely out of himself!

R. L. Gregory remarks that, "An entire world may be created and mistaken for reality." However, there are hazards. "Stimulation by bright flashing lights can be an unpleasant experience, often leading to headache and nausea." Even the flashes of a television screen may be "dangerous for people with a tendency to epilepsy."

People are to be a part of the psychic environment, participate in it, perhaps even manipulate it. Such an environment is animate and not static. It prods the senses and the psyche, if not overpowers them. Some feeling of space will be created, allowing more room for the spirit to soar. There will be a partial if not complete journey out of reality. The environment will be more personal.

What is to be done? To begin with a couple of simple principles, conceive of people in terms of space within an interior. Seymour Evans, a New York lighting engineer, talks of space lighting. Theatrical downlights and spots are proposed to throw light patterns into which and out of which people can move. These could be of different tint and might have the cheerful effect of a walk through the woods on a summer day. Evans also mentions the buried beam, which more or less conceals a bulb of lamp and creates light within space that comes from no apparent source.

For human participation, a well placed projection lamp having a point light source will cause a person's shadow to strike a nearby wall. He can thereupon use his arms and body in any antics he wishes. Even more dramatic, General Electric Dichro-Color spot lamps in red, green, and blue can be placed close to each other or in the form of a cloverleaf and directed toward a wall or curtain. As people move about, their shadows will be in rainbow hues, although the total blend of the three spots will, for additive reasons, form a fairly neutral white light.

Psychic lighting has not, of course, come out of the laboratories of illuminating engineers. On the contrary, the psychedelic artist has scouted lighting equipment and created inventions of his own. Recently there has been a collaboration of scientists and artists in an effort to see what can be done jointly. There are new vehicles to exploit, polarized light, the laser beam, nuclear radiation.

There is beauty and attraction in colored *light*, not to be found in pigments and dyes or even fluorescent materials. Colored light has a celestial quality; it seems pure, luminous, and radiant. It is seen at its best in near or total darkness, and here it gets all the more attention. Abstract color and abstract form have existed in what have been called "color organs" for quite a while. In the eighteenth century a Jesuit, Louis Bertrand Castel, wrote about music and color. "Can anyone imagine anything in the arts that would surpass the visible rendering of sound, which would enable the eyes to partake of all the pleasures which music gives to the ears?" He developed a "Clavessin Oculaire" which apparently projected colors through transparent tapes.

Color organs were subsequently devised by D. D. Jameson (1845) and A. Wallace Remington (1893). In America Bainbridge Bishop (1877) blended colors with organ music and sold one of his instruments to the eminent P. T. Barnum. Mrs. Mary Hallock-Greenwald (1926) won a gold medal in Philadelphia and "played" colors on a screen along with a symphony orchestra. Of greatest fame, however, was Thomas Wilfred and his Clavilux (1921). He gave color concerts throughout the United States and looked upon abstract, mobile color as an art form in itself. Another pioneer was Tom Douglas Jones whose Chromaton offered an unending and ever changing array of flowing abstract forms and colors. Still another innovator, Cecil Stokes of California, around 1945, produced a series of Auroratone films which were used in veterans' hospitals to treat psychotic patients. Abstract colored motion pictures, accompanied by the singing of Bing Crosby and the orchestral music of Andre Kostalanetz, found good success in breaking through emotional and mental barricades and making patients "accessible" to psychiatric care. All these men beheld visions, which LSD and psychedelic art were later to seize upon and expand to larger dimensions.

As one artist declares, "We try to vaporize the mind by bombing the senses." Stroboscopic lights tend to stop motion or at least slow it down like old movies. Lights shift, change, flow, assume weird and pulsating forms. Sounds blare. Even perfume may be added. Attempts are made to destroy space through the use of illuminated floors, mirrors, spots of light that seem as far away as stars. People are "turned on" without drugs. Electronic gadgets convert sound waves to colors. The old, Gothic fascination of the stained glass window is resurrected, but with the images far more brilliant and stirring.

Psychic lighting has become part of the modern discothèque. It has entered advertising, displays, entertainment. While the glitter and dissonance of it may drive oldsters out into the open and back into their conventional homes, it motivates people to act together, and it remarkably breaks down barriers between them. Though there may be a certain wildness and lack of control today, psychic lighting may become one of the most important, functional, and rewarding contributions to the artificial environment of the future.

One of the first total psychedelic environments was that exhibited in New York at the Riverside Museum in 1966 (see Color Plate II). In a small cavelike structure vibrant colors and strange images of gods, demons, and humans were projected overhead, while the occupants, lying on a turntable, slowly revolved. All in sight was color, form, and motion. The responses to the museum visitors who were thus "turned on" is not recorded, and perhaps no psychological or other study was made. But this writer feels very sure that anyone suffering from severe melancholia or dejection could be shaken out of the mood — at least for a spell.

In a splendid article for The New York Times Magazine (May 12, 1968), Eleanore Lester has described other such psychedelic environments. In one, called "Fanflashstick," a minidiscothèque is constructed of clear plastic film, and within it are flashing colors, whirling balloons and confetti, flickering strobe lights, and raucous tape noises. In the space are invited a number of persons, young and old, all of them with their senses assaulted to near-mad limits. According to the creators, Gerd Stern and Michael Callahan, the electronic enclosure "expands the consciousness and intensifies the perception. . . . The sensory bombardment tends to break down old patterns." Stern declares: "Now, lights have a way of making us time-conscious. The flashing allows us to make pattern discriminations within time. The flash of the strobes freezes the movements of people, and people really do move very differently from one another. You should see the difference in the way the Fanflashstick looks when it's filled with basketball players, and how it looks when it's filled with girls from a small Catholic college."

The day is rapidly approaching, when even the most conservative and austere environment will be endowed with more life and vitality through the introduction of psychic lighting in some form or other. In an office, factory, school, daylight sources, plus some ultraviolet, may be utilized for a good part of the day. Yet for psychological and emotional reasons, other lights in other intensities and tints may be programmed: warm light in the morning, increased intensity and whiteness as the day progresses, "complexion" lighting at coffee breaks or during the noon hour, pink or orange light again at dusk.

Perhaps for those with neurotic or even psychotic troubles, "color therapy" of the psychedelic type may be prescribed, along with harmonious music or comforting sounds. As the practioner of psychosomatic medicine knows only too well, a high percentage of human ailments — from asthma to ulcers, the hives, stomach cramps, heart flutter, shortness of breath — all too often begin in the mind. The afflicted mortal sinks to brooding over his misery and his condition grows worse.

If light and color can help to save him from himself, draw him out of his despondency, get him agreeably involved in the world around him and the people in it, then light and color by all means should have an essential place in a new era of illumination for man-made environments to come.

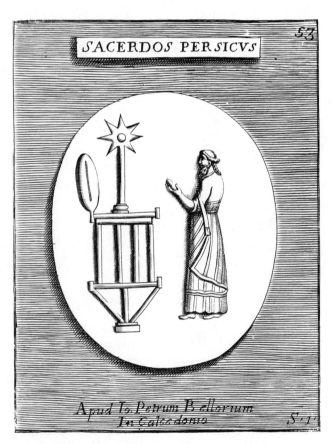

Zoroastrian priest and the mysteries of the cosmos.

CHAPTER TEN

Light vs. Color Value

There are two vital principles to remember in applying colors to interior environments. The first of these is that of A. A. Kruithof, mentioned in Chapters 4 & 8. It is normal—and best—*for the tint of a light source to be warm in quality at low levels of intensity and cool in quality at high levels.* This concerns what is usually referred to as normal artificial light, from incandescent to the white and blue-white sources of modern times. Never use cool white light at low levels, and avoid light that is too yellowish or orange at high levels. And don't forget this!

Now for the second principle: *Be aware of the fact that color values (degrees of brightness) will appear in their true identity only at reasonable and high levels of light intensity, not at low levels.*

Illumination creates and destroys space. It changes the aspect of things in the world in endless ways. Space is never empty, nor can it be conceived as being filled with nothingness. Darkness is a positive factor in human perception, not a negative one.

Space and illumination are perceived in terms of the objects and surfaces seen within them. The world seems broad and wide under bright light. In dim light the world of space crowds in like a great tent. Poets and people say that night falls, that it approaches stealthily, that it shrouds the day. The truth, of course, is not that darkness comes in, but that light fades out.

Under bright light space is readily defined, distance can be easily determined, forms appear round and three-dimensional, while details, colors, and color variations are all clearly seen. When light grows dim, however, space seems to contract, distances cannot be effectively judged, forms tend to flatten out into silhouettes, details are lost, and colors and color values undergo radical transformation.

As a scientific point, R. L. Gregory remarks that "The cones [on the retina of the eye] are most sensitive to orange, while the rods are most sensitive to green." Further than this, under bright illumination yellow occupies the region of highest visibility in the spectrum. Under dim light, highest brightness is found for blue-green. Yet where the eye is dark-adapted — as at night — color discrimination is difficult, if not lost entirely. The cones of the retina, of course, operate almost exclusively in average or bright light, while night vision is largely the function of the rods of the eye.

On this matter of illumination, space, and colored surface, when a person enters a planetarium, he will be quite conscious that a structural dome is overhead. When the lights go out, the dome will seem to vanish, and stars and planets will float in infinite space. Today in the psychedelic environment, space is often caused to disappear or retreat through the strategy of a black overhead, mirrors, point light sources that make vision beyond them impossible.

While the psychedelic effect may be wanted, at times it may occur when not intended. Here is an example. A symphonic hall is painted a deep navy blue, a sober and perhaps appropriate color in itself. However, when lights are dimmed, perception loses all grip on the color. It disintegrates, so to speak, and loses its identity. This becomes disturbing to the audience, for in dim light the environment loses clear definition and character.

There may be nothing intrinsically wrong with navy blue, but for this dark color to be seen in its true beauty a great deal of light is needed. Without such light it is meaningless. Moreover, black has similar odd characteristics. No black surface absorbs all light. One is confronted with the strange fact that black needs light to appear black; and the more light that shines upon it, the blacker it will become — though it actually will be reflecting more light.

The great majority of architects, interior designers, and others who specify color for buildings, seem to be unaware of certain definite occurrences that take place *in the apparent brightness or value of colors* as illumination levels are varied from dim to bright. This is a phenomenon noted by many students of vision and was given special attention by the German psychologist, David Katz.

Despite the wonders of color constancy (the persistence of vision in seeing genuine color qualities under widely different conditions of light), the values of color undergo shifts when exposed to different degrees of light intensity. By the term *value*, the author refers to apparent brightness or reflectance.

Consider the following points:

(1) As long as the eye is able to see, a white surface will always appear white — from under a fraction of a footcandle to high into the hundreds of footcandles.

(2) In complete dark-adaptation, the eye loses *all sense* of color. This is because the cone endings of the retina, sensitive to color, grow dormant, and seeing is taken over by the color insensitive rods.

(3) However, because near-darkness is seldom encountered in a decorative problem, the phenomena of complete dark-adaptation may be set aside.

(4) Looking at a scale of gray values from white to black, the relationships of the steps will remain normal — one to the other — for *all* illumination levels above 25 or 30 footcandles.

(5) Below 25 or 30 footcandles, however, there will be a pronounced contraction.

(6) This is because, as illumination grows dim, all deep colors tend to "melt" together in value or brightness, if not in hue.

(7) For example, under 30 or more footcandles of light, the mid or medium point (value) on a neutral scale will be judged as a gray having a reflectance of about 20 percent. Such a gray, under good light, will appear to be visually half-way between white and black.

Under 20 footcandles, the mid-step will require a reflectance of about 25 percent to appear half-way between white and black.

At 10 footcandles, the mid-step will require a reflectance of about 30 percent.

At 5 footcandles, the mid-step will require a reflectance of about 40 percent.

And at 1 footcandle, the mid-step will require a reflectance of about 45 or even 50 percent.

(8) In brief, as light grows dim, (a) the gray scale becomes shorter and shorter, *but from the bottom up;* (b) all the dark tones below any judged mid-step will tend to blend together and appear alike in value or brightness. White alone will hold its constancy.

Many practical lessons may be learned from this phenomenon or principle. At the bottom, for example, in very dim light the true values of the dark colors will be lost more or less completely. The U. S. Navy at one time used black for the walls of submarine conning towers and combat information centers where near darkness was necessary during battle operations. This standard has been changed to a medium green, and for a clear reason. When the eye is dark-adapted, *any color reflecting 20 percent or less will appear black.* So why use black? After all, battle practice is infrequent on a naval vessel. Most of the time the lights are on. Personnel, instead of being exposed to a black coffin of an interior, can be surrounded by a pleasing green — with no sacrifice of functionalism in the color treatment of the interior.

There are other morals to be drawn from the principle being discussed here. For example, it is wholly incongruous to pick colors in bright light and expect them to appear the same under dim light. Again, if the environment is designed for soft light (a living room, a cocktail lounge, an exclusive restaurant, an enclosed sitting or rest area), there is little sense in using dark colors. Dark colors, in fact, may "fall apart" and grow muddy. If the eye of an occupant in a dimly lit room is to sense and appreciate the colors of the decor in walls, floors, furnishings, *no color with a reflectance of less than 10 or 15 percent should be used.* Anything deeper may be meaningless — if not ugly because of the inability of the eye to perceive it clearly.

There is still another factor to bear in mind. In establishing space relationships in a building, either for the exterior or interior, there is a wholly natural sequence of perspective. White, black, pure hues, and deep shades will all appear near the eye. In what artists call aerial perspective, as colors shift or fall back into the distance, that which is dark increases in value; that which is light in value softens a bit — and all things eventually fade into a medium light gray. Color schemes can be planned to feature this phenomenon, using strong colors and strong contrasts for near elements, and grayish colors and weak contrasts for far elements. In the old days when multistory buildings were given egg and dart or other decorative cornices, this ran contrary to the facts of aerial perspective. Detail cannot be seen from a distance, so why put it twenty, thirty, or more stories into the air!

CHAPTER ELEVEN

The Use of Color on Exteriors

The eight color schemes in Color Plates III and IV display the use of different effects and materials in unusual ways—not within homes, where color is often desired, but on large-scale public, private, and commercial buildings.

Color is rarely found on the exteriors of modern buildings in modern cities. In America, in particular, architects have generally emphasized original and unique building designs at the expense of color. As a result, as Frank Lloyd Wright once remarked, all tend to look alike in their attempts to be different. Europeans have often followed master plans utilizing traditional colors.

In ancient times exterior color was the rule rather than the exception. The temples, shrines, mosques, pyramids, and palaces of Egypt, Asia Minor, Greece, and South and Central America were richly adorned with color. In many instances their beauty vies with and often surpasses that of later centuries. While lavish *interiors* were created during the Renaissance and after, *exteriors* for the most part abandoned artificial in favor of natural color.

Some scholars have attributed the decline in the use of exterior color to two factors. First, ancient cities were often located in warm, dry climates where inclement weather did not rapidly deteriorate man-made pigments and coatings. Second, with the Reformation, ostentatious design was criticized as "pagan." Color was sensuous, vulgar, and even sacrilegious. While images of saints within churches could be adorned with colorful garments and jewels, those outside the church must be carved of pure stone or marble.

In the western world numerous state capitals and public buildings duplicate Greek architectural elements but without the colors that embellished the originals! Although the ancient Greek could admire brightly colored statues, today the use of color is more or less inconceivable in any sculpture that pretends to true elegance—it must be marble, stone, or bronze!

Frank Lloyd Wright (1869–1959) was the champion of natural color. Color Plate III–A shows his Arizona headquarters, Taliesin West, which remains a school of architecture and a tourist attraction. Wright utilized only natural materials. He rejected the use of paint, resorting to a sand-finish coating where necessary. His one favorite color—used on his letterhead—was a terracotta red, and he at times used it as a stain for exposed wood or steel.

Wright was ingenious in his use of concrete, cast-concrete blocks, and steel cantilevers. Color was denounced as the concern of "interior desecrators." The pylon shown in Color Plate III-A is made of colorful natural stone, which was as far as he would go. Much of his architecture, particularly homes, featured low horizontal lines and projecting eaves— and was designed *to blend into* the natural environment. Taliesin West well epitomizes this goal.

Should architecture fit into an environment or stand out bravely from it? There are two schools of thought, and one may argue effectively either way. The natural, fit-in position has a loyal champion in Jean-Philippe Lenclos of France, who differs from Wright in his dramatic use of natural local colors.

Lenclos is noted for his designs for industrial facilities, factories, cranes, tanks, and smokestacks. Even more remarkable, however, is his approach to town housing. He collected regional samples of natural earths and clays and developed palettes based on them for use in mass housing. He has also incorporated the colors of the sky, water, and vegetation. When the colors of his palette (drawn from a specific region) are applied in paint finishes and other building materials, the final result looks appropriate and harmonious.

Plate III-B shows a color plan developed by Lenclos for a housing development at Le Vaudreuil in France. He collected samples of earths indigenous to the region, including clay, sand, soil, loam, slate, and stone, from which a palette of about 25 color swatches was prepared and matched in paints and building materials. (Sky colors were added.) This method of using color seems well suited to rural and suburban regions, less suited to crowded urban areas with nary a tree in sight.

Charles Eduard Jeanneret, Le Corbusier (1887–1965), also of France, unlike Wright or Lenclos, used color in architecture as a factor in itself, with less regard to natural or environmental conditions. He was a famous painter, architect, and writer. He based his compositions on sound geometry, admiring Cubism but objecting to any decorative tendencies. His architecture has had a great international influence. He devised a host of new construction methods, such as modular systems for mass production. He designed villas, workers' housing, chapels, a national capital (in Punjab, India), and a visual-arts center (at Harvard).

For the apartment house shown in Plate III-C, Le Corbusier used semaphore-flag colors—vivid red, yellow, green, and blue. The effect is sophisticated, timely, and appropriate to the geometric style of the building. For the interior of a monk's chapel Le Corbusier applied massive areas of bright red, dark blue, gold, and tan paint to concrete, leaving the impressions of the wood grain quite evident. In both cases there was no pretension to cover up the stark and bold use of color.

Le Corbusier had a great fondness for color: "Color could bring us space. It contributes elements of extreme physiological potency to the architectural symphony." If Wright believed that man was natural and should respect natural materials, Le Corbusier traced his roots back to the very beginnings of civilization: "Color is not descriptive but evocative; ever symbolizing. It is end and not means. Considered from a certain point of view, folk art survives the highest civilizations. It remains a norm, a kind of measure the standard of which is natural man—the savage, if you will." And the savage loved color!

Plate III-D shows a Brazilian chapel by Oscar Niemeyer, an admitted admirer of Le Corbusier. Again, color is used in concert with design as an architectural form. Would a chapel of natural stone be any more appealing? Niemeyer is notable for his plans for Brasilia, the new capital of Brazil constructed in previously uninhabited territory. This commission brought him world-wide fame. His chapel, which utilizes cool blue tones, is meant to stand majestically in contrast to nature, not to harmonize with it. It is meant to represent the human expression of spiritual and religious feelings.

The German Bauhaus was a revolutionary and functionally sound school that established new modes of building design and construction totally lacking in furbelows. With the demise of the Bauhaus in 1933, America welcomed such men as Walter Gropius, Marcel Breuer, Mies van der Rohe, and Herbert Bayer, and architecture in this country witnessed a radical change. Strangely enough, in the fine arts the Bauhaus produced some of the most outstanding creative work in color, the products of such painters as Wassily Kandinsky, Paul Klee, Josef Albers, Johannes Itten, and others, while in architecture the geometric concepts made little allowance for it. Concrete, brick, stone, and glass are all honestly utilized, but there is a definite paucity of ornament and color. The criticism can certainly be raised that black or bronze structures, unadorned, with dark, light-absorbing glass, behind which are black or brown Venetian blinds are immense sepulchers fit for dead rather than living human beings.

Plate IV-A shows the library of the National University of Mexico, designed by Juan O'Gorman, which is part of a complex of modern buildings constructed under the direction of Carlos Lazo. O'Gorman's mosaic murals depict in realistic as well as abstract and symbolic fashion the story of Mexico from ancient to modern times.

Mexico is not unfamiliar with brightly decorated architecture. Precedents were established centuries ago in the magnificent and mysterious pyramids, temples, and structures of the Mayan, Toltec, and Inca civilizations, in which abstract and symbolic design, coupled with bright color, were applied freely. In effect, O'Gorman's library reflects the architecture, art, and color expression of ancient Mexican culture, the beauty of which ranks with that of Egypt, Asia Minor, and Greece—and has a similar color spirit.

Plate IV-B shows facades of buildings in the General Motors Technical Center at Warren, Michigan. This immense undertaking, backed by George C. Booth, was originally inspired by the talents of the Finnish architect Eliel Saarinen (1873–1950), who designed major buildings at the Cranbrook Academy near Detroit. It was taken over by his even more talented son, Eero Saarinen, who at the age of 38 completed the project and thereby gained recognition as one of America's leading architects. He had a meteoric career. He designed strikingly original buildings at Yale, Vassar, the University of Chicago, the American embassies at London and Oslo, and the soaring TWA air terminal in New York.

The G.M. Technical Center features huge facades in glazed brick, colored in bright red, rich blue, and golden yellow, with expanses of fenestration in between. The structures thus tend to look different from different directions. Through this simple but highly effective device, color is put to impressive use without employing embellishment. Saarinen's distribution of color in these end-wall treatments was new and original and it well deserves emulation in the future.

Plate IV-C shows a blast furnace at the Jones & Laughlin steel mill in Cleveland, designed by Faber Birren. Due to the effects of coal, coke, smoke, and soot, equipment was normally painted black—not for appearance but for protection. Today, with the introduction of oxygen and electricity, the grimy days and black shrouds can be replaced with more colorful raiment.

To some eyes, blast furnaces and steel mills are august to behold. In black they may seem ominous, but in color they take on a grotesque majesty. While air pollution no longer was an overriding factor, inert iron ore, which has a brownish tan color and tends to settle everywhere as harmless dust, had to be taken into account. Samples of this dust were studied in terms of how it would affect the appearance of colors. Three basic hues of metal-protecting finishes were developed, a golden tan (the color of the dust itself, used mostly for storage sheds), a terracotta or henna red, and an olive green, all of which were not seriously altered by the iron-ore dust. The bright yellow was originally specified for oxygen lines and had to be retained. Where the original black was austere and funereal, associated with heavy air pollution, the scheme in golden tan, terracotta, olive green, and yellow brought an attractive dignity to a practical and essential industry.

Plate IV-D shows a sectional view of the famous (and notorious) Centre Beaubourg in Paris, popularly known as the Museum Georges Pompidou. This spectacular building, with most of its structural elements and utilities exposed and brilliantly colored, may seem incongruous and grotesque indeed in one of the most consistently beautiful cities anywhere in the world. Why were non-French architects chosen?

The design of the Centre Beaubourg was opened to competition, and the architects who submitted plans remained anonymous. The decision went to an Englishman and an Italian, Richard Rogers and Renzo Piano. And what eventually saw the light of day in Paris brought astonishing reactions. If the Centre Beaubourg is disliked by some purists, no one can doubt its success, if such success is to be measured in terms of popularity. It was "packed" the day it opened and has been "packed" ever since.

Why the bold color? According to Rogers, "A strong influence on our work is the way in which color is used as a safety factor in the coding of industrial environments and machinery: steel plants, refineries, tractors and cranes. We believe that buildings are machines." Rogers questioned "classical monochromatic elegance" and wanted to expose the "works" of the Centre with industrial colors "used for marking hazards and identifying certain equipment." Because most of the building was constructed of steel, it demanded protection from the elements; and, if finishes were required, they might just as well be brightly colored.

Perhaps this colorful adornment of architecture echoes the similar brave use of primary hue so prevalent in centuries past. Perhaps in the world of tomorrow architecture will forsake elegance for vitality and let color play the dynamic role that it has always held within the psyche of man.

CHAPTER TWELVE

Office Color Plans

The seven chapters that now follow are meant to offer information on the application of color to offices, factories, schools, hospitals, motels and hotels, stores, food service. These refer to color standards in the specifications list. The author has been able to draw from wide experience in all these fields, and, in addition, to propose colors and effects that will assure the best of scientific practice.

To begin with offices, decoration here is hardly a matter of esthetics or personal taste — at least in principle. In the castle of the home, individual taste has every right of expression, for color is emotional in content and means different things to different mortals. In business, however, the direction needs to be less subjective than objective. People in an office are supposed to get things done and not merely sit around to enjoy themselves. It is fallacious to assume that because color is appealing and attractive, it is conducive to enjoyable labor. Indeed, for the very reason of its strong impact, it may, when not properly applied, distract from work, interfere with tasks, and actually make seeing difficult and fatiguing.

Unfortunately, much office decoration today is far from functional. Interior designers and architects tend to express personal views and feelings, and having used a certain scheme in one building, see the need to use something else in another. This often leads to a style or fashion approach and to office interiors that look more like recreation or living areas than working spaces.

A technical approach to color is not complex. A manufacturer of office furniture needs to decide upon an ideal color for a desk and desk top. If his product were sold for home use, he would have to cater to the whims of the consumer and be aware of color trends. He could, of course, make his desks in a variety of hues — and most office furniture manufacturers do so. Yet to perform a service to the buyer of office equipment, he wishes to make his color choice in every way as functional as the dimensions and mechanical features of what he produces.

With appropriate attention to advice from ophthalmologists and lighting engineers, he selects a warm gray with a reflectance of about 30 percent. This is similar to specified color Pearl Gray. The reasons are as follows: such a color is neutral and nondistracting. It strikes a neat balance in brightness between white and black. As a background, this tone quality helps to keep the eye of the employee at a uniform and comfortable level of adjustment and to "cushion" visual shock as a worker glances from light ceilings to dark floors, or from bright details in his environment to deep ones. As evidence that he has done a good job, the desk manufacturer can refer to a series of ophthalmic tests which indicate that his optical gray reduces the rate of eye blinking, effects less fatigue in retinal and convergence reserve, and is judged pleasant as a sort of extra dividend.

If an architect or designer objected to gray on esthetic grounds (this is less likely among businessmen), at least one lesson would be learned. In this particular instance, the factor of brightness is more important than that of color. Therefore, any soft hue reflecting about 30 percent of light would do equally well. With one visual condition set and proved, the emotional quality can be given wide latitude.

After all, to establish an ideal and comfortable environment in offices — on walls, ceilings, and floors, as well as on furniture and equipment — brightness is more significant than hue. And because it is, the designer or architect may express himself as he likes — just so he does not put the eyes, emotions, and bodies of people under undue stress. As examples, it would be wise for him to avoid too much use of white (which happens to be fashionable at the moment). White may make it difficult for a worker to concentrate on anything else. It may constrict the pupil opening of the eye, fog vision, introduce tiring glare, and handicap clear vision of vital work tasks. None of these reactions has to do with taste or personal opinion; they involve physiological responses which can't be argued away on esthetic grounds.

Deep colors, on the other hand, may cause details to be glare sources, open the pupil of the eye too wide, and hence lead to visual fatigue. It would be "functional" to maintain the ceiling bright for good light reflection, to keep walls between 40-60 percent reflectance, floors, furniture, and equipment above 20 percent (up to 40 or 50). An occasional end wall in a softer hue is both esthetically and physiologically desirable. (Colors on end walls, incidentally, originally came out of the industrial field and set the vogue for homes.) The end wall color relieves monotony and provides a welcome area for temporary rest and relaxation of the eyes (see the Munsell notations).

The great advantage of color is that it is spontaneously pleasing. Because its brightness can be "engineered" at will, office design can be given infinite variety. Principles can be followed, while other rules are avoided, to create environments which not only are casually attractive but which contribute to human comfort and efficiency over hours, weeks, and months of occupancy.

With an eye on the Munsell notations supplied, here are a series of definite recommendations. It will be recalled from earlier chapters that color and brightness can have two different visual, physiological, and emotional effects. Where there is high brightness and warm color, attention will extend outward to an environment, and this reaction may be favorable for the performance of muscular tasks. On the other hand, where there is lower brightness and cooler color, the environment will be less distracting, human attention will be directed inward, and the reaction here will be favorable for more exacting visual and mental tasks.

Good colors for general offices (see Color Plate V) will be found in Soft Yellow, Coral, and Chartreuse, for a warm effect.

Also appropriate and more refined would be Sandtone and Beige.

Oyster White would be cooler, and so would light Green and Aqua.

To produce some variety, major walls could be painted Sandtone, and end wall and freestanding columns could be in Soft Yellow, Rose, Pale Gold, Fern Green. Or, the major walls could be Oyster White, with end wall and freestanding columns in Soft Yellow, Colonial Green, Smoky

Blue. Brilliant colors are not recommended as accents for fear of distraction.

In private offices and conference rooms more tolerance may be exhibited, although extremely dark colors are not advised. Walls could be in Sandtone, Beige, or the softer Pale Gold, Colonial Green, Smoky Blue, Taupe. A more striking effect would be to have Oyster White on three walls, with the accent end wall in Terra Cotta, Old Gold, Avocado, Emerald Green, Turquoise, Sapphire Blue. Different offices, of course, may use different hues. However, deep or strong colors should never be put on window walls; they are best placed on walls in back of desks, or on walls faced by personnel.

In rest rooms, Rose, Pale Gold, Fern Green, Colonial Green, Smoky Blue are all suitable; or wall coverings in these tones, with or without patterns, could be considered.

For corridors, Oyster White, Sandtone, or Beige may be used for the wall on one side, with the opposite wall in a luminous color such as Pumpkin or Bright Yellow. Here visual stimulation would be quite permissable and desirable.

Different colored doors can be used anywhere in offices, and a good range of colors would consist of Terra Cotta, Old Gold, Avocado, Emerald Green, Turquoise, Sapphire Blue.

Movable partitions would appear best in colors comparable to Oyster White, Sandtone, Beige, with brighter hues on other walls.

For food service areas see Chapter 16.

In office equipment and furnishings, a point has already been made regarding desk tops. The desk bodies themselves can be in different hues, but soft tones are best, such as Pale Gold, Fern Green, Colonial Green, Smoky Blue.

Carpeting is preferred on the light side and in soft, pale tones of beige, gray, or green. Furniture upholstery colors are more effective when they contrast with walls. Beige, brown, and orange complement green (or the reverse); blue appears bright with gold, red with aqua or turquoise. Academic theories of color harmony can be disvaluated and set aside for good, reasonable judgment. The standards noted on the table may serve as guides. Respect these and be wary of those colors that are not included (orchid, purple, vivid yellow-green).

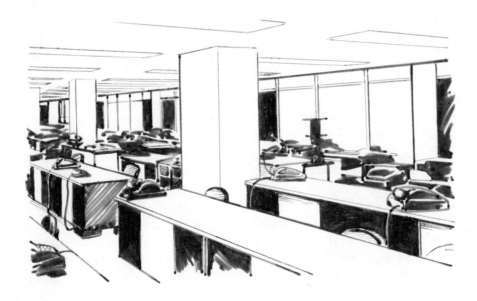

A NOTE ON COLOR SPECIFICATIONS

The first edition of this book included two charts with 72 mounted chips of colors. Direct reference was made to these by specific color names. Today, however, in this newly revised and updated work, the high cost has prohibited the inclusion of the charts. However, their equivalent Munsell notations have been recorded and are given below. Through this happy device, the color names have been retained. The Munsell identifications may be accurately determined by referring to the Gloss Edition of the *Munsell Book of Color*, the most widely and universally known method of color notation—which is conveniently available in many libraries, colleges, architectural and interior-design firms, advertising agencies, commercial organizations, scientific laboratories (devoted to color), and private collections.

Approximate light reflectances for each color and notation are given in brackets. The names used for the colors are descriptive in themselves and may suggest standards for the reader. Reference may also be made to the Color Plates of this book, in which many of the mentioned colors are illustrated.

OYSTER WHITE, N 8.5/ (67%)
SANDSTONE, 10YR 9/1 (79%)
BEIGE, 10YR 8/2 (59%)
CORAL, 10R 8/4 (59%)
PEACH, 5YR 8/4 (59%)
SOFT YELLOW, 5Y 9/4 (79%)
CHARTREUSE, 5GY 9/4 (79%)
LIGHT GREEN, 10GY 9/2 (79%)
AQUA, 2.5BG 9/2 (79%)
LIGHT BLUE, 10B 8/4 (59%)
ROSE, 5R 7/4 (43%)
PALE GOLD, 2.5Y 8/4 (59%)
FERN GREEN, 2.5GY 7/4 (43%)
COLONIAL GREEN, 5G 7/2 (43%)
SMOKY BLUE, 5PB 7/4 (43%)
TAUPE, 5Y 7/2 (43%)
PEARL GRAY, N 8/ (59%)
TERRACOTTA, 7.5R 6/4 (30.4%)
OLD GOLD, 2.5Y 6/4 (30.4%)
AVOCADO, 10Y 6/4 (30.4%)
EMERALD GREEN, 5G 6/4 (30.4%)
TURQUOISE, 5BG 6/4 (30.4%)
SAPPHIRE BLUE, 7.5B 6/6 (30.4%)
VERMILION, 7.5R 5/12 (20%)
FLAMINGO, 5R 7/8 (43%)
PUMPKIN, 5YR 7/8 (43%)
BRIGHT YELLOW, 5Y 9/6 (79%)
MAROON, 5R 3/6 (6.6%)
WALNUT BROWN, 7.5YR 3/4 (6.6%)
FOREST GREEN, 10GY 4/4 (12%)
NAVY BLUE, 10B 3/6 (6.6%)
CHARCOAL, N 4.5/ (12%)
FIRE RED, 2.5R 4/10 (12%)
VIVID ORANGE, 2.5YR 6/14 (30.4%)
VIVID YELLOW, 10YR 8/14 (59%)
VIVID BLUE, 10B 5/10 (20%)

OPAL PINK, 2.5YR 8/2 (59%)
ADAM GRAY, 5YR 8/1 (59%)
VERNON GRAY, 10P 8/1 (59%)
FRENCH GRAY, N 7.5/ (50%)
CHALK GREEN, 10GY 8/2 (59%)
POWDER GREEN, 5GY 8/2 (59%)
POWDER PINK, 2.5R 8/2 (59%)
FLESH PINK, 2.5YR 8/4 (59%)
WASHINGTON GOLD, 5Y 8/2 (59%)
PALE CITRON, 10Y 8.5/4 (67%)
OPAL BLUE, 7.5B 8/2 (59%)
POMPADOUR BLUE, 10B 7/4 (43%)
ROSE POMPADOUR, 2.5R 6/6 (30.4%)
POMPEII RED, 7.5R 5/16 (20%)
VERNON ROSE, 5R 7/4 (43%)
ROSE BEIGE, 10R 6/2 (30.4%)
GOLDEN OCHER, 7.5YR 7/8 (43%)
EMPIRE YELLOW, 5Y 8.5/10 (67%)
GEORGIAN GOLD, 5Y 7/6 (43%)
ORIENTAL GOLD, 7.5Y 6/4 (30.4%)
APPLE GREEN, 7.5GY 8/4 (59%)
SOFT GEORGIAN GREEN 5GY 7/4 (43%)
DEEP GEORGIAN GREEN, 5GY 5/4 (20%)
DARK OLIVE, 5GY 4/4 (12%)
MALACHITE GREEN, 2.5G 6/6 (30.4%)
EMPIRE GREEN, 2.5G 5/8 (20%)
GREEN ROOM, 2.5G 4/4 (12%)
GEORGIAN BLUE, 5BG 5/4 (20%)
SÈVRES BLUE, 5B 7/4 (43%)
DELLA ROBBIA BLUE, 7.5B 5/6 (20%)
BLUE ROOM, 2.5PB 5/4 (20%)
WEDGWOOD BLUE, 2.5PB 5/6 (20%)
FRENCH LILAC, 10PB 7/4 (43%)
VICTORIAN MAUVE, 2.5P 4/4 (12%)
PERKINS VIOLET, 5RP 6/10 (30.4%)
RED ROOM, 5RP 5/8 (20%)

CHAPTER THIRTEEN

Industrial Plants

The applied science of functional color is greatly concerned with problems of visibility, acuity, and ocular fatigue. It deals with visual conditions encountered in factories, offices, schools, hospitals, and it seeks to perfect these conditions through the specification of tried scientific principles.

As a brief historical review, functional color had its beginning in the mid-twenties of this present century. At that time studies were made in hospitals to lessen glare and improve the vision of the surgeon. To accomplish this, new techniques were worked out whereby the degree of fatigue could be measured by instrumental means. Results were achieved in the control of brightness and hue that quite definitely established the value of color in aiding human efficiency and well-being.

As adapted to hospitals and schools — and later to industrial plants and offices — "color conditioning" was applied to increase production, improve quality of workmanship and normal skill, reduce "seconds" and "rejects," cut down accident frequencies, raise standards of plant housekeeping and machine maintenance, reduce absenteeism, and improve labor morale.

Despite automation these days, human eyes are obliged to undertake constantly more difficult tasks. In fact, the automation process with its intricate mechanisms and multitudinous cards, records, and films, puts eyes under severe strain and leads to problems not encountered a few decades ago. And color has to a large extent come to the rescue.

Where the eye is taxed, where seeing is attempted under severe tension or strain, a number of physiological and psychological reactions are to be observed. The eye itself may increase its rate of blinking. There may be a dilation of the pupil after several hours, even though the intensity of light may not change. Power to hold the eyes in convergence, to distinguish small brightness differences, to focus for a clear image, may be reduced. There may be a reduction in sensitivity on the outer boundaries of vision; the eye may be less able to see clearly in the peripheral areas of the retina.

Most of these effects will disappear if the eyes are rested. However, prolonged abuse may result in permanent damage. The pathology of eyestrain has been treated at length by Ferree and Rand. The chief cause of distress is usually traceable to high and disturbing brilliancies in the field of view. Such brilliancies may constrict the pupillary opening and hence deprive the eye of sufficient light to see clearly. As a consequence, there may be an unhealthy congestion within the blood vessels of the eye. In young persons these congestions may actually cause elongation of the eyeball and thus nearsightedness. As Ferree and Rand conclude, there may be disturbances in the mechanism of the eye, the iris, and lens. There may as well be damage to the retina itself, which may take the form of inflammation or detachments. "The eye has grown up under daylight. Under this condition only three adjustments have developed, and indeed only three are needed: the reaction of the pupil to regulate the amount of light entering the eye and to aid the lens in focusing the light from objects at different distances, and accommodation and convergence to bring the object on the principal axis of the lens and the image on the fovea. . . ." These adjustments tend to be coordinated. When they are separated, trouble is encountered. High brightness in the field of view, if isolated from the task, may cause disruption. The eye will thereupon struggle to set things right. *This striving to clear up its vision by ineffectual maladjustments is the cause of what is commonly called eyestrain.*

M. Luckiesh has written: "A visual task is inseparable from its environment. . . . High visibility, ease of seeing and good seeing conditions are overwhelmingly the result of good brightness engineering." Eyestrain thus finds its master not solely in illumination, nor in proper diet and medical care, but also in color and the ability of color to add efficiency and comfort to seeing. It is obvious, for example, that if great brightness extremes exist within the field of view, the pupil of the eye will be forced to undergo constant changes of adjustment. Areas too light in color may set up psychological distractions and defy concentration on other objects and tasks. "The eyes often adjust themselves to a bright peripheral object notwithstanding the fact that the attention is directed elsewhere." (Luckiesh). Seeing would be as difficult under this condition as the attempt to hear a speaker while someone kept ringing a bell.

It is quite possible to set forth ideal brightness specifications for factory and office conditions. Ceilings, almost without exception, should be white. A colored overhead will not only quench valuable light, but it may distract attention upward and away from jobs at hand. White overheads will be essential to the efficiency of natural and artificial lighting systems.

Upper walls (generally to a line level with the bottom of roof beams or trusses) should have a reflectance between 50 and 60 percent (if floors and equipment are on the dark side), or between 60 and 70 percent (if most areas and surfaces in the interior are, or can be made, fairly light). Wall brightnesses higher than 70 percent seem to be allowable only where the most perfect and modern lighting system is installed and accompanied by pale floors and equipment — or for unimportant spaces such as storage, where critical seeing tasks are not performed. It must not be forgotten, however, that bright walls are not flattering to human appearance.

If a dado is required to conceal stains, the color tone should reflect not less than 25 percent and perhaps not more than 40 percent. Floors should reflect at least 20 percent, if this is practical. Machines, equipment, desks should have a reflectance factor between 25 and 40 percent, lighter when the floor is light and deeper when the floor is dark.

These ratios and percentages have been successfully applied in numerous plants and thus have the benefit of widespread trial and research.

Certain refinements are also to be introduced. Window sash ought to be white or a light tint to lessen contrast with outside brightnesses. Machinery may be highlighted with a pale color, such as buff, to reflect more light at important parts and concentrate the attention of the worker. In numerous fine seeing tasks, background shields may be constructed to (1) reflect light and provide immediate contrast with materials, (2) confine the vision of the worker and hold eye adjustments relatively stable, (3) blank off shadows or movements in the distance, and (4) give the worker a better sense of isolation. Normally such shields should cover from 45 degrees to 60 degrees of the visual field.

End wall treatments in medium tones also have widespread application. Where most workers may be engaged at difficult eye tasks and may be oriented to face in the same direction, the wall ahead may be colored in a pleasing tint, having a reflectance of from 25 to 40 percent. The end wall will help to overcome an unfavorable constriction of the pupil. Upon glancing up, it will afford relaxation rather than the stimulation of glare. It will likewise relax the strain of prolonged convergence and be psychologically pleasing and restful. Here again is a principle widely and successfully employed in industry.

Referring to Color Plate VI, it is logical to use "cool" colors such as Light Green or Aqua, where the working condition exposes the employee to relatively high temperatures. Conversely, "warm" tones of Peach, Soft Yellow, Beige are suitable for softening up a vaulty or chilly space and to compensate for a lack of natural light.

In purely casual spaces, such as washrooms, rest rooms, and cafeterias, lighter and cleaner hues may be used. In view of average color preferences, Light Blue becomes ideal for facilities devoted to men, and Coral for facilities devoted to women. In stairwells and corridors, usually deprived of natural light, bright tones of Soft Yellow are effective. In storage areas, white is best and will make the most of existing lighting installations.

Where critical seeing tasks are performed, however, and where distractions are to be avoided, the best colors to use are soft variations such as Pale Gold, Fern Green, Colonial Green, Smoky Blue, Taupe. Large, vaulty spaces may be enlivened with Peach or Beige over all walls, or Soft Yellow over end walls. Gray machinery highlighted with a buff on important parts and working areas will prove effective. A medium gray is also ideal for unimportant elements such as bins, racks, shelving. One must remember that color is more compelling than neutrality. Hence, if it is strategically applied, it can make order out of chaos, distinguish important from unimportant elements, and help the worker in his mental effort to concentrate on his task. In theory as well as practice, the purpose of color is not so much to "inspire" the worker; too much of this attitude may lead to distractions and irrelevancies. On the contrary, color becomes integral with the task, not foreign to it. Improved efficiency and relief from fatigue become automatic, because the human eye can see more easily, with less strain. Color is chosen to fit in rather than stand out. It contributes to better visibility and to an agreeable and cheerful frame of mind.

Finally, a color code for safety should be mandatory in the factory or industrial plant. One developed by this writer is now used in the shore facilities of the U. S. Army, Navy, and Coast Guard. It is organized generally as follows (see Color Plate VI).

Vivid Yellow (or yellow and black bands) is standard for marking strike-against, stumbling, or falling hazards. It is painted on obstructions, low beams, dead ends, the edges of platforms and pits. Being the color of highest visibility in the spectrum it is conspicuous under all lighting conditions and well adapted to the above purposes.

Vivid Orange is standard for acute hazards likely to cut, crush, burn, or shock the worker. It is painted around the edges of cutting machines and rollers. On the inside areas of machine guards and electric switch boxes, it "shouts loudly" when such devices are removed or left open.

A brilliant green is standard to identify first aid equipment, cabinets for stretchers, gas masks, medicines, and the like.

Fire Red is reserved entirely and exclusively for the marking of fire protection devices. It is painted on walls behind extinguishers, on floors to prevent obstruction, on valves and fittings for hose connections.

Vivid Blue is standard as a caution signal. The railroad industry employs it to mark cars which should not be moved. In factories it is placed as a symbol on equipment, elevators, machines, tanks, ovens, etc., cut down for repair. It may be used on switch control boxes as a silent and unobtrusive reminder for the worker to see that his machine is clear before he operates it.

White, gray, or black are standard for traffic control and good housekeeping. They are used for aisle marks, and painted on waste receptacles. White corners and baseboards may be used to discourage littering and to stimulate the sweeper to dig into corners.

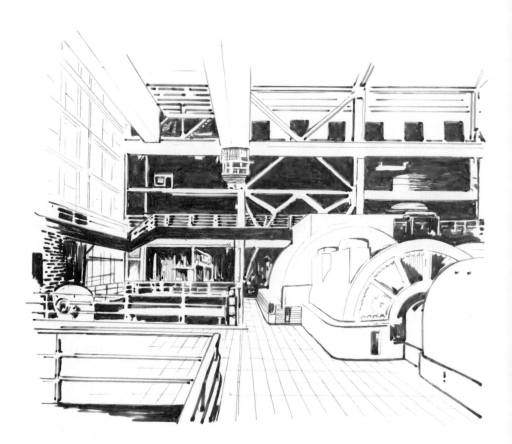

CHAPTER FOURTEEN

Schools

Carefully planned experiments by psychologists have well proven that modern principles of color applied to schools will improve in a striking way the scholastic performance of school students, especially noteworthy in the earlier years. A well designed environment not only facilitates learning new subject matter, but reduces behavioral problems. Then, too, there is the vital purpose of protecting eyesight and safeguarding the welfare of young and old alike.

There is little argument but that functional color has an abiding place in the school plant. However, overemphasis on "beauty" and "fashion" may defeat the true purpose of color and detract from that functional dignity which should prevail in the school field. Color for the sake of color is hardly practical.

The overwhelming advantage of functional color is that it is purposeful. It is concerned with measurable things, and since this is so, one can predict with considerable accuracy what is likely to happen if certain definite principles are followed. Personal opinion and even whims, which so often complicate color choice, may be set aside for sound technical practice.

The causes of fatigue and eyestrain are well known: glare; continual adjustment to areas of conflicting brightness; prolonged convergence on near tasks; poor visibility. When conditions are poor, the scientist may use instruments to measure the rate of blinking, muscular tension, the dilation of the pupil of the eye, and the reduced sensitivity of the retina.

If, through good illumination and correct choice of color, better results are attained, one may be assured that a good job has been done, and the facts will speak for themselves.

From the standpoint of *vision*, several fundamental principles have emerged in recent years. It is obvious, of course, that the eye needs ample light to see clearly. But once this illumination is made available through the efficient manipulation of natural and artificial light sources, the ideal environment demands equal attention to the color and brightness of the surroundings.

For example, light colors reflect more illumination than dark ones. Too much brightness, however, may handicap vision (a) by creating unfavorable glare; (b) by unduly constricting the pupil opening of the human eye; and (c) by interjecting a disturbing psychological and visual "pull" away from books and tasks.

Most authorities today seem to be in agreement on two points. First, brightness ratios in the general field of view (walls, floor, furniture, equipment) should be fairly uniform.

Second, the school environment (ceiling excepted, which should be white or off-white for good light reflection and the reduction of shadows) should be painted in colors that reflect between 50 and 60 percent. Fur-

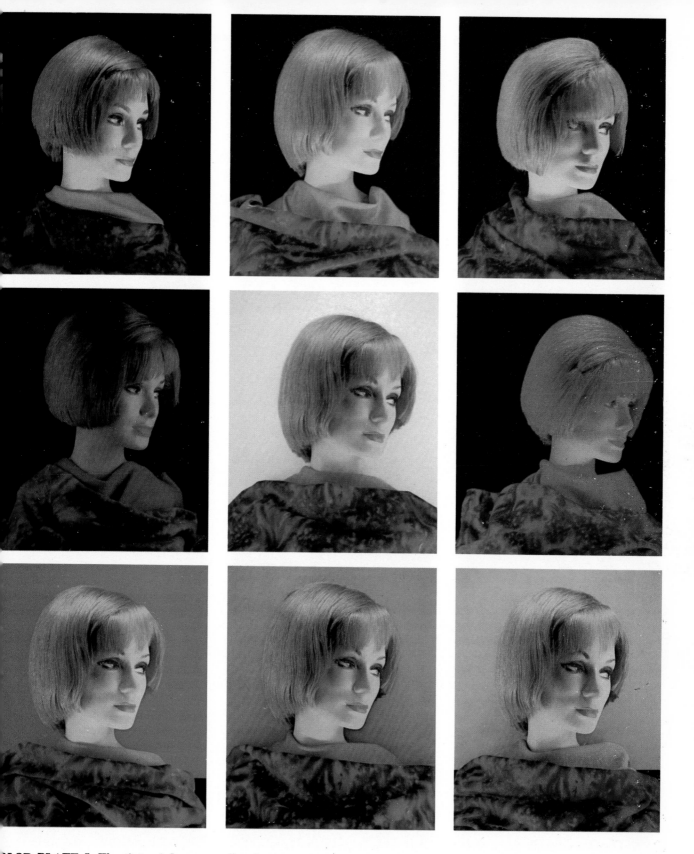

COLOR PLATE I. The tints of fluores-
nt light sources influence the appear-
ce of human complexion. Upper left is
aylight with a color temperature of
out 6800°. The effect here is bluish.
pper center is Duro-Test Optima with
temperature of about 5500°. Here the
effect is more or less neutral. Upper right
is Cool White (about 4300°), and the
effect is slightly on the yellow-green side.
Middle left is Warm White (3000°) comparable to candlelight. Middle right is a
definite pink illuminant. Middle center
and all three bottom illustrations are
Duro-Test Optima and show effects of
different colored backgrounds: white, red,
turquoise, lime green. The white ground
tends to dull complexion; red tends to
drain it of pinkness; lime green tends to
turn it purple; while turquoise (blue-
green) is most flattering.

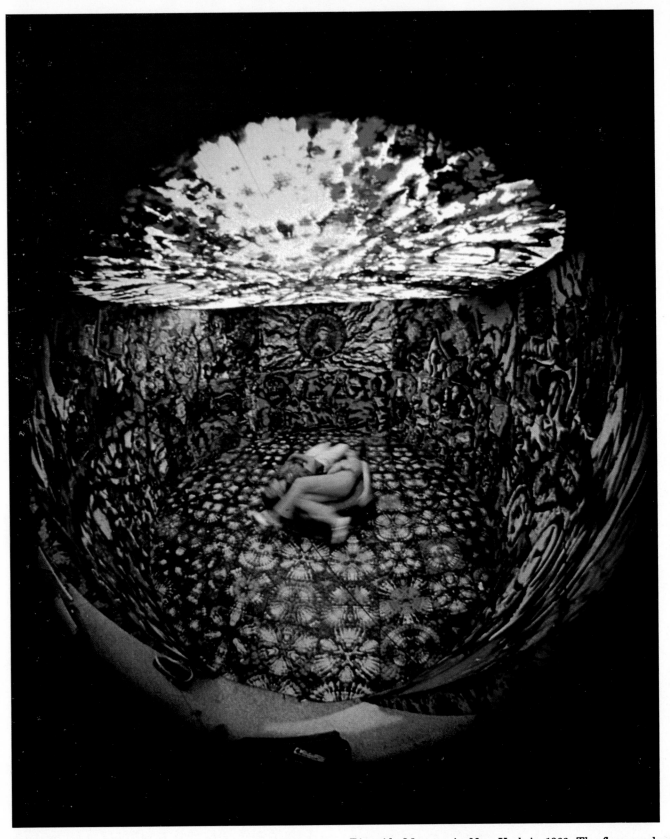

COLOR PLATE II. This is an early historic example of a psychedelic environment. Developed by a creative group called USCO (The US Company), it was exhibited at the Riverside Museum in New York in 1966. The floor revolved slowly amid a surround of gods, demons, and humans. (Photography by Yale Joel, Life Magazine, © Time Inc.)

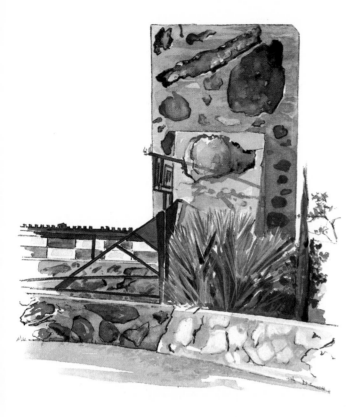

A. Taliesin West, Frank Lloyd Wright.

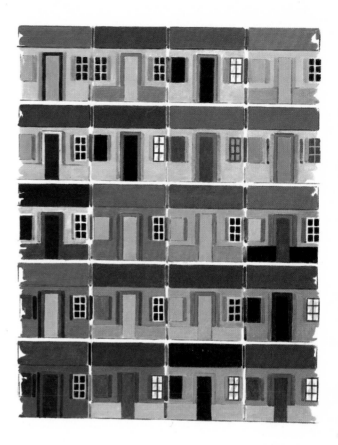

B. Color planning, Jean-Philippe Lenclos of France.

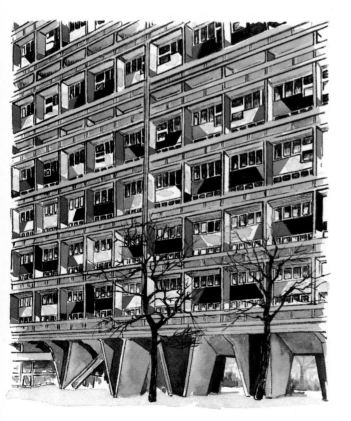

C. Berlin apartment, Le Corbusier.

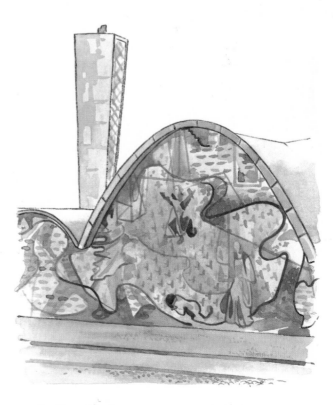

D. Chapel in Pampulha, Brazil, Oscar Niemeyer.

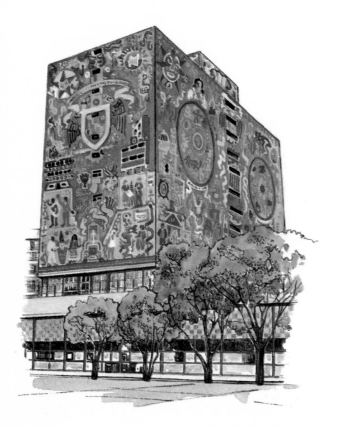

A. Mural, library, National University, Mexico, Juan O'Gorman.

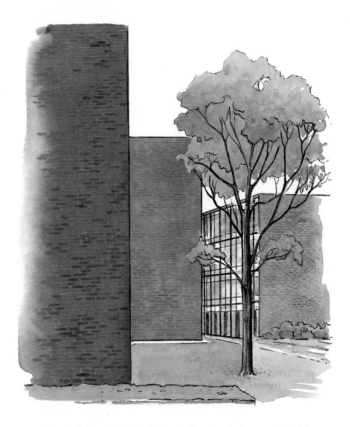

B. General Motors Technical Center, Warren, Michigan, Eero Saarinen.

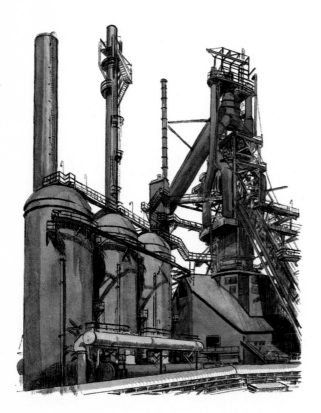

C. Cleveland blast furnace, Jones & Laughlin Steel Corporation.

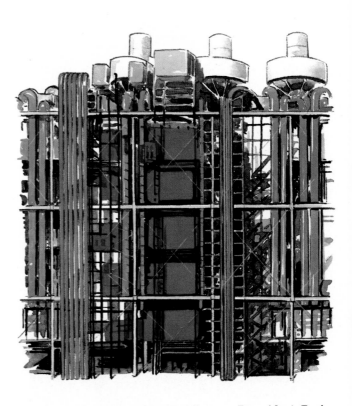

D. Centre Beaubourg (Museum Georges Pompidou), Paris, Richard Rogers and Renzo Piano.

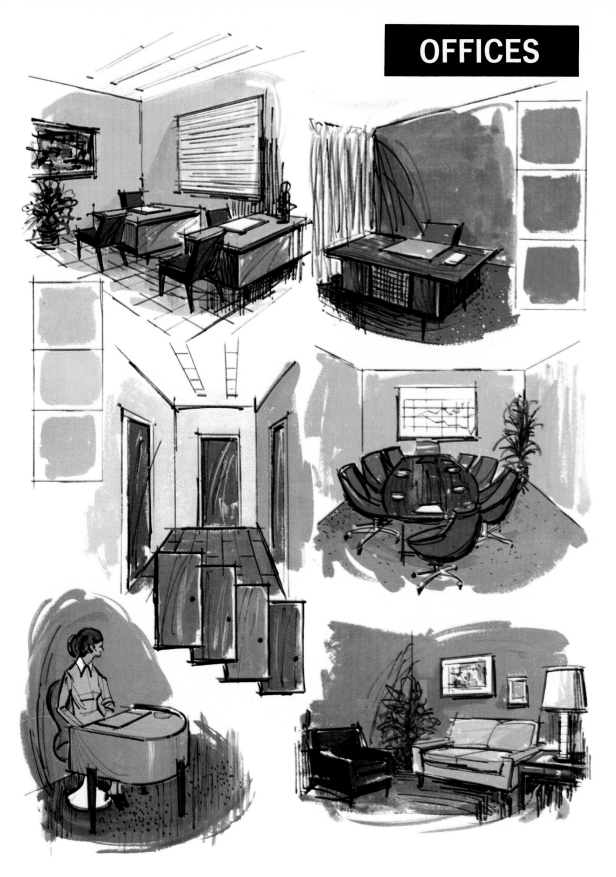

COLOR PLATE V.

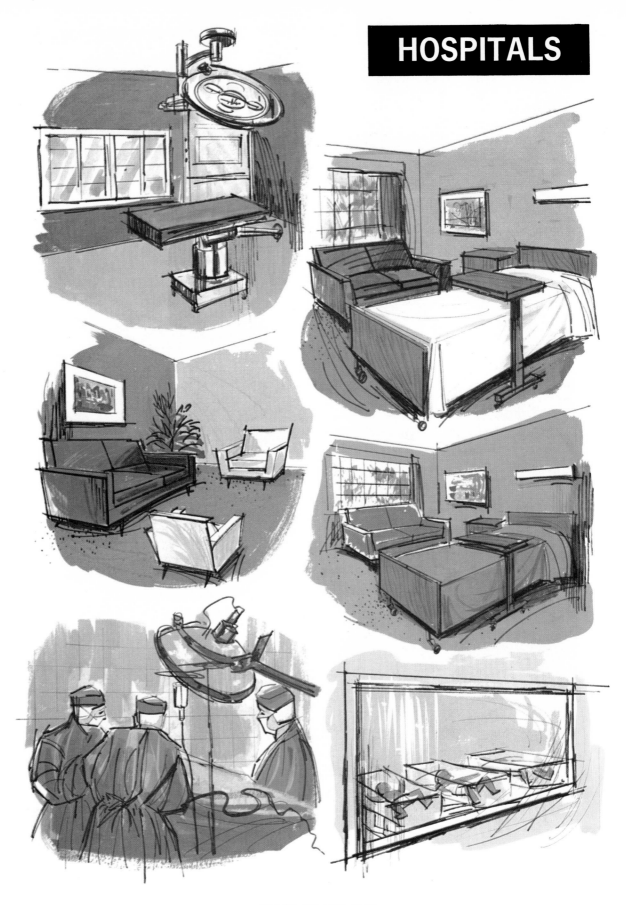

COLOR PLATE VIII.

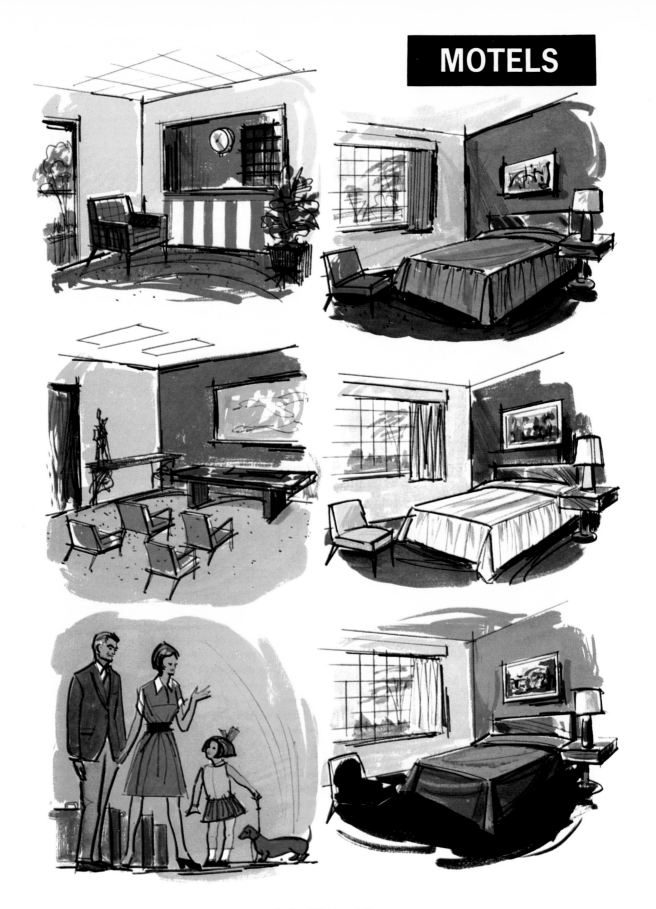

COLOR PLATE IX.

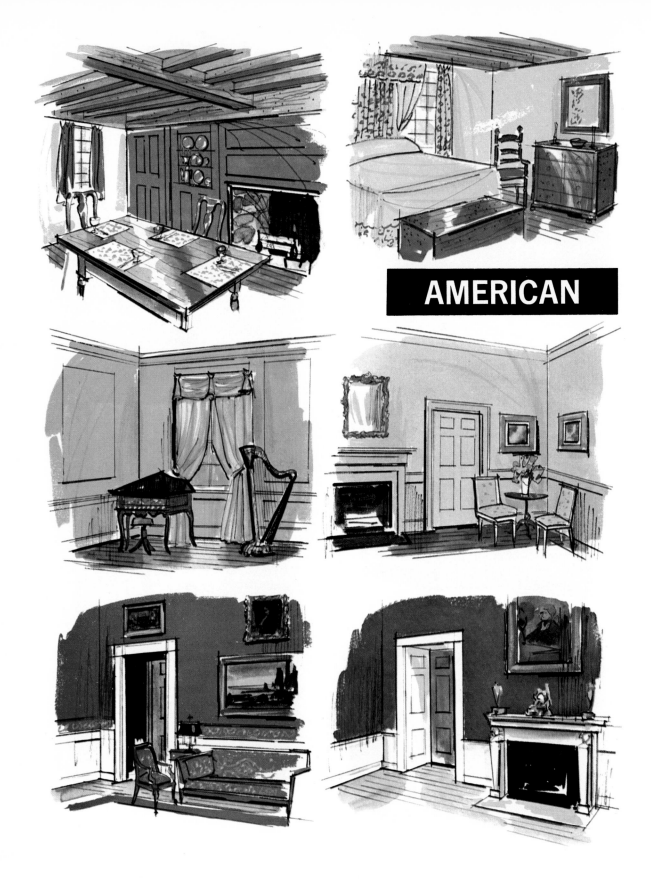

AMERICAN

COLOR PLATE XVI.

niture, equipment, and walls may reflect between 30 and 40 or 40 and 50 percent for some relief and practical resistance to soiling and abuse. Assuming a uniform distribution of illumination, the maximum ratios of brightness difference (30–60 percent) would be 2 to 1 (or 3 to 1 at the most between a furniture finish of 30 percent reflectance and a white ceiling of 90 percent reflectance).

Where the brightness ratio lies within 5 to 1, seeing is "smooth" and unencumbered, and average school tasks may be comfortably performed.

Floors should reflect from 20–30 percent — the actual range of unstained natural wood. On the other hand, desks and equipment should range in reflectance from 25–40 percent; brighter finishes with higher reflection are only acceptable where all other areas of the room can also be made correspondingly high in reflectance.

Irrespective of details, color is an important experience in life. It is needed in the school field, not only for its charm and beauty but to provide normal emotional outlets. A gray or buff world has little outward appeal. It tends to lead to subjective moods, to inner tension and monotony. Color, on the other hand, provides release, excitement, pleasure. And because most psychological troubles may be traced to inner workings of the mind, the stimulation of color is good tonic to the senses and good distraction from fears and apprehensions.

There is enough evidence available today to give the color plan real purpose and direction (see Color Plate VII). First of all, the bright environment, the warm colors—Soft Yellow, Coral, Peach —will have a diverting effect. Because visual and emotional interest will proceed outward, the bright, warm color scheme becomes highly appropriate for kindergartens, elementary grades, places of relaxation and diversion. Because virtually all children are born extroverts, the dynamic setting invites an outward release of feelings and emotion—and because of the release, nervousness and tension tend to be dissipated.

Whereas brightness and warmth pull attention outward, softness and coolness of color have a reverse effect. With ample illumination, the walls should be toned to Chartreuse, Light Green, Aqua, and the passive effect of the surroundings will permit better concentration. It will not impose upon the pupil's need and desire to direct his attention inward rather than outward. Hence, cool colors become appropriate for upper and secondary grades, study rooms, and the school library.

End wall color treatments are particularly appropriate to schools. In classrooms where students are oriented to face in one direction, the wall so faced can safely be toned to great advantage and comfort. The best practice is to use a tint like Oyster White, Sandtone, or Beige for side and back walls, and to have the front wall in medium colors, such as Terra Cotta, Old Gold, Avocado, Emerald Green, Turquoise, Sapphire Blue. The advantage here is that the colorful end wall will (1) relax the students' eyes upon looking up from their tasks; (2) add greater visibility to the teacher and to the lessons or educational materials displayed; and (3) break up monotony by giving the classroom a different appearance from different directions.

Bear in mind that the critical use of the eyes or brain is upset by distractions — glare, sharp color, noise, movement. Where the effort is to come from within, the environment must be subdued, so it will not set up an annoying competition. Aquas and greens accomplish this by causing the surroundings to recede and allowing the child to devote himself to the exacting demands of thought and contemplation.

Interior decoration as a purely aesthetic approach to color is seldom as appropriate as practicability and functionalism. It is good standard practice to use white for *all* ceilings, both for consistent appearance and to reflect an abundance of shadow-free illumination. Again, trim may be a uniform light or medium light gray or beige — doors, door frames, window sash, baseboards, lockers, cabinets, shelving, bins, and miscellaneous equipment. A special blending trim color for every wall color may be desirable in a home, but in a school it complicates the color plan and fails to tie together the general facilities of the school plant. One common trim color not only looks appropriate but saves cost in painting and paint inventory.

As for other school facilities, libraries, rest rooms for teachers, school offices, these could well be in subdued tones of Pale Gold, Fern Green, Colonial Green, Smoky Blue.

Cafeterias should be in Peach, Coral, Rose, Pumpkin, Flamingo. All of which are cheerful and "appetizing."

The gymnasium, shops, manual training, and domestic arts rooms probably are best in luminous tones of Soft Yellow, Peach, Beige. Locker rooms and dressing rooms in Coral will reflect a flattering light. Laboratories are well considered with tones of Colonial Green or Pearl Gray. The auditorium may be one of several hues, although Rose, Pale Gold, or Fern Green are suggested because of their warm and friendly tones.

School buildings are for the populace at large and should seek democratic rather than sophisticated values. Colors such as green, blue, yellow, coral, and red have well known appeal, as revealed by psychological research in color preference. They have impulsive and spontaneous charm recognized by most persons. To venture afield from these known qualities of pleasure in color is to contradict the direct and unprejudiced purposes of education.

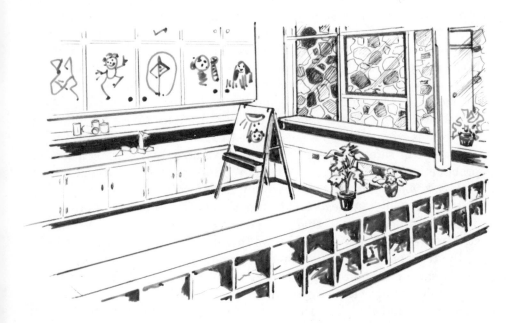

CHAPTER FIFTEEN

Hospitals

One of the problems with color in hospitals is that it has such a strong emotional content. In viewing it, people experience subjective impressions which vary according to human temperament. This confuses the issue of color and often clouds a logical and practical attitude towards it. There seems to be no middle course — the spectrum is either magical or impotent, and opposing forces are lined up.

The psychological sciences have not had an easy time gaining the recognition they hold today. Psychosomatic medicine, however, has finally impressed the point that a high percentage of human ills may be traced to psychological tensions, anxieties, and fears. If pathological disturbances result, no cure is effective unless the mental condition is attended along with the physical one. Here is where color is significant and where its role in hospital planning and decoration is important. Man is responsive to his environment and is affected by it. If there may be no direct therapy in color, there is much indirect psychotherapy that could be applied.

Enough research has been conducted in recent years to warrant a fairly rational specification of colors in hospitals. Unfortunately, because human reactions to colors are emotional, clinical data are not easy to gather, and facts are difficult to quantitate. Nonetheless, tendencies are strong enough in certain directions to justify a number of general if not specific conclusions. Here are a few of them.

As has been discussed in this book, brightness and vividness of color *tend* to arouse autonomic functions, blood pressure, heart, and respiration rate. Cortical activation is increased, and the organism tends to direct its attention outward toward the source of stimulation. Dimness and softness of color *tend* to have reverse effects and to invite repose. Autonomic functions are retarded and, with the environment passive, there is less outward distraction and more inner relaxation.

It is commonly admitted today by many psychiatrists and clinical psychologists that color has one simple but clear effect: its emotional impact tends to lead to outwardly directed attention. In other words, it is diverting and pleasing. This in itself is good for any patient, for it may offer some relief, even if minor, from inner tensions. It has the same influence as any agreeable sensation, and in this sense it is at least conducive to recovery.

Still omitting any specific therapy for color, it would seem from the above generalities that a hospital color plan can be built upon intelligent elements and not left to mere chance or personal feeling. Above all, the plan should be individual to the hospital. Surely it should not attempt to impose anyone's personal views as to what constitutes beauty. As a matter of fact, beauty should be a by-product of utility.

On this latter point, there are some uses for color in the hospital which do not essentially concern beauty or emotion. In surgery, for example, the development of artificial light sources of high intensity more than a decade ago led to problems of glare, which were to a large extent resolved in the use of special tones of green and blue-green tile and other wall materials. Such application of color reduced brightness in the field of view, built up better visual contrast, complemented the reddish tint of human blood and tissue, and thus aided the acuity of the surgeon's eyes. The factor of appearance was wholly incidental.

In accommodations for patients, color control for comfortable vision is a primary requisite, before emotional factors need to be considered. Beds should be located with windows to one side rather than full ahead. It is a known fact that the eye can adjust itself almost constantly to differences in brightness, *if the major field of view is involved.* This condition is found in nature. What it cannot accept with comfort is strong contrasts *at one and the same time!*

Thus, in private rooms and wards, the hospital plan more or less begins with the establishment of a soft and uniform field of view. Ceilings should perhaps be tinted because of the supine position of the bedridden guest. Wall areas and floors should be soft in tone, with a reflectance between 40 and 60 percent. Furnishings and draperies should not be too pure in hue or too pronounced in design. Brilliant reds, yellows, and blues may be "pretty" enough for well persons, but they are unduly impulsive and may grow monotonous to a confined patient. Yet in parlors, solaria, and recreation areas, more freedom can be permitted — and is desirable for an interesting change of pace.

It is obvious that, as reason is brought to bear on the hospital color plan, variety automatically results, not as an end in itself, but as a result of purpose and function. This is the way things should be, for the hospital environment will be designed in a way that is individual to its needs and rightfully adapted to the high purposes of medical care.

As for precise color choice, psychological prescriptions are more complex to write than strictly visual ones. Color in its subjective effects is quite personal, and likes and dislikes will vary. There are many who will say they "love" certain hues and "hate" others, and reasons for such views will be vague. If there can be no answers, at least it becomes sensible to take whatever research and evidence has been assembled from competent sources and to use them as a guide, if not as a rule.

In overall studies of color reactions and associations, three "maxima" of appeal are found in blue, red, and green (and their tints and variations), and "minima" are found in orange, purple, and other intermediate hues. Simple logic would suggest that certain colors like yellow-green and purple lack universal appeal and at the same time are anything but "healthy" looking. There are better colors than these for hospitals.

Blue is something of an exception. While it may be desirable as a decorative accent, large areas of it tend to have a cold and bleak look. Being sharply refracted by the lens of the eye, blue causes a near-sighted condition that disturbs some persons. However, it finds a less objectionable variation in tones of aqua and turquoise.

For a visualization of hospital effects see Color Plate VIII. In patients' accommodations, fairly soft tones are better than "sharp" ones for reasons of greater subtlety and refinement. If warm, bright colors *tend* to be exciting and to draw attention outward, they seem desirable for convalescent patients. Here there would be a good reason to consider moderate tones of Coral, Peach, and Soft Yellow. These would create subjective feelings which are more or less positive in nature. On the other hand, if cool, subdued colors *tend* to be subduing and to inspire a more relaxed mood, they become suitable for chronic patients. The hospital palette may thus further include tones of Light Green and Aqua (avoid Chartreuse).

More subdued tones are also suitable. In the surgical suite and operating room, Turquoise is more or less requisite. This is complementary to the pinkish tint of human blood and tissue and is almost universally used today in operating room garments, surgical caps and masks, operating table towels and sheets. Recovery rooms can be the same Turquoise or the lighter Aqua.

Private rooms could be in Rose, Pale Gold, Colonial Green — in addition to the pastels listed above (avoid Fern Green). The nursery could be Coral.

In X ray and physiotherapy, Aqua is ideal. Various clinics, treatment and examining rooms could be in Coral, Peach, Light Green, Aqua.

Solaria and visitors' rooms could be Soft Yellow. Or, end wall treatments could be used, having Oyster White, Sandtone or Beige for three walls, with the accent wall in Terra Cotta, Old Gold, Emerald Green, Turquoise, Sapphire Blue — or bright colors such as Flamingo or Pumpkin.

Offices and laboratories could be in Oyster White, Sandtone, Beige, Pale Gold, Colonial Green, Taupe — or Pearl Gray, where good color discrimination is necessary.

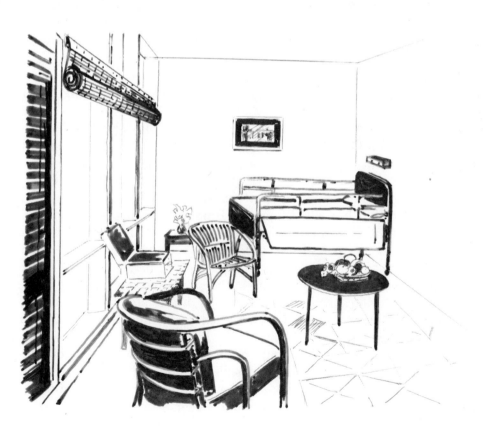

CHAPTER SIXTEEN

Motels and Hotels

The decoration of hotels, motels, and resorts involves many of the factors encountered in stores. Therefore, similar colors may be considered applicable. The public expects much color these days — and it has good taste. As in the case of stores, exceedingly high style ventures may not accomplish what management expects. Color for the sake of color holds no particular merit, for, while a drab environment is emotionally discouraging, too exotic an effect may lead to rejection. The appeal of color is at unconscious levels, and people are sensitive without really knowing why. If you surround human beings with colors they innately dislike — and seldom if ever buy — you automatically sponsor distaste. An interior designer can, of course, do as he wishes and be as contrary as he or his client wants, but why take the chance? After all, there are plenty of striking and compelling hues to which people respond spontaneously and favorably.

In bedrooms, parlors, suites, any number of principles may be followed. Here Oyster White, or Sandstone, or Beige is perfectly suitable for any or all parts of a hotel or motel and is an excellent foil for brighter hues. In bedrooms, it may be applied to three walls, with the forth wall in a deeper hue—Terra Cotta, Old Gold, Avocado, Emerald Green, Turquoise, Sapphire Blue.

For a varied and well balanced color plan, consider the following (refer to Color Plate IX).

In bedrooms use any light colors such as Coral, Peach, Soft Yellow, Chartreuse, Light Green, Aqua, Light Blue. Or, combine a light neutral color with end walls in deeper tones, as just described. Or, use tone-on-tone effects: Coral with Terra Cotta, Soft Yellow with Old Gold, Chartreuse with Avocado, Light Green with Emerald Green, Aqua with Turquoise, Light Blue with Sapphire Blue. Also consider Flamingo, Pumpkin, Bright Yellow. Where the deeper color is used for one wall, give it a generous area—such as the back of beds—but never use it on window walls.

For the lobby and for public spaces, the sky is more or less the limit. However, to introduce modern trends in color, use Oyster White as a base or key note. Variety can then be achieved by adding bright and rich colors on columns, across end walls, in alcoves.

In the psychological sense — and quite successful in store decoration as well — variety is the spice of life. Its visual and emotional actions tend to draw attention outward and to evoke a definite (if moderate) stimulation. It invites movement and traffic and a keen interest in the environment.

However, if for some reason a more reserved and "cozy" atmosphere is required in a hotel or motel, the overall effect can be subdued and use can be made of the medium or deep colors. This might apply to luxury type suites, to parlor and meeting rooms. Be careful, however, not to repeat the vogue of the fifties, in which deep greens made caverns of many a hostelry. If medium or deep colors are preferred, contrast them with light ceilings, columns, floors, furnishings, to give the eye a full sense of color values and not leave it lost in darkness. Good large area colors for a modified effect are found in Rose, Pale Gold, Fern Green, Colonial Green, Smoky Blue, and Taupe.

Colors as deep as Maroon, Walnut Brown, Forest Green, Navy Blue are not advised over large wall areas for average hotel lighting conditions—lest trouble be encountered with the principle described in Chapter 10 on Light vs. Color Value.

In theatres and meeting rooms, the surrounding spaces may require specifications such as given above. The theatre itself requires a measure of care. Colors too light, such as white, may have very strong reflections. Remember that, regardless of the intensity of illumination, white is always seen as white, due to the phenomenon of color constancy. Stage productions or moving pictures may flood side walls near the stage or screen with unfavorable and disturbing brightness if white is employed here.

Colors too deep, on the other hand, may get completely "lost" in dim illumination for reasons of color constancy, given in an earlier chapter. A fair appearance may exist with the lights on, but when the lights are down, the dark-colored walls may fade out into a "nothingness" and give the interior a weird atmosphere.

Good colors for theatre interiors, therefore, are in the medium range. Suggested are Old Gold, Avocado, or the muted Pale Gold, Fern Green, Colonial Green, Smoky Blue. Not to be too severe, some trim or details — such as the overhead and the undersides of balconies — may be in lighter tones of the same hues. Or, the trim and overhead may be in neutral Sandtone or Beige.

If different colors are wanted on different walls, the two sides of the auditorium should be the same, while a different color (or two different colors) may be applied to the area surrounding the stage or screen and to the back of the theater.

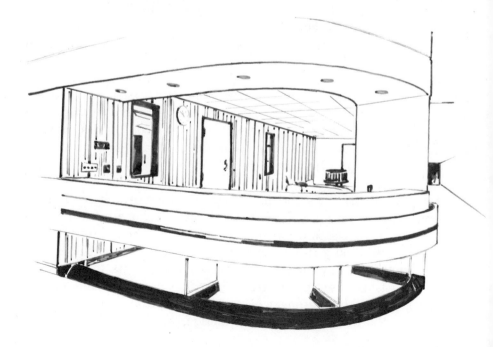

CHAPTER SEVENTEEN

Shops and Stores

A well coordinated store — in terms of color — is primarily concerned with the wants and desires of the American public. As every experienced retailer understands, good merchandising is not a matter of whim or personal opinion. In consumer goods *right* colors sell in profitable volume, while *wrong* colors lie dormant in unsold and costly inventories.

In store decoration every retail outlet is a "package" which must be sold to the public. Good colors appeal on sight, invite traffic, draw from competition, and otherwise serve economic (not merely artistic) ends in modern business. If the store *appearance* is drab, if it is too old or too high fashion, the customer may turn on his (or her) heel and shop elsewhere.

As for illumination, Kruithof's principle should be respected. At low levels of illumination, warm light is best and most normal. In merchandising warm light is ideal for products such as home furnishings — because homes by and large are dimly lighted (usually with incandescent sources).

Not to overlook customer appearance, warm fluorescent or incandescent light becomes almost mandatory for personal products, such as women's fashions and cosmetics. Here also the warm light should have a modeling effect in highlight and shadow and should not be too flat. Bear in mind that while cooler lighting may give colored products a realistic appearance, it may at the same time make the customer look unnatural. Sometimes it is far better to flatter the customer than the things she is buying. For if *she* looks bad, she may not buy anything at all!

In impulse merchandising, package goods and the like, really bright light, and cool light, is well prescribed. Personal appearance may be of secondary importance; by giving life and brightness to the merchandise, more of it may be sold.

It would seem good policy in average retail stores to let the general illumination be warm for the customers' benefit. Cooler sources more like natural daylight may then be specified over merchandise, when accurate color discrimination is necessary. In food stores daylight light may enhance vegetables, and pinkish light may add richness to meats. However, too much overall cold light must be avoided; it won't be liked.

As for the color or walls and fixtures, there are research reasons and functional reasons why certain colors are better than others. To begin with, the most appreciated colors in the psychological sense are blue, red, and green. (Yellow may also be accepted for its high visibility and compulsion.) These primary hues thus become good accents for signs, end walls, and displays. They appeal on sight, for they are universally enjoyed by all age levels and by persons of all races and cultural backgrounds.

Because of the need for impulse attraction, wall colors in stores and shops can be on the clean, clear side. For example, Oyster White could be used as a general sequence color. End walls, walls around elevators, and freestanding columns could then be introduced in bright colors—perhaps Flamingo for women's departments, Sapphire Blue for men's, Pumpkin or Bright Yellow for housewares, drugs, and merchandise to be bought on sight. A color such as Turquoise becomes practical for walls and backgrounds in the sale of many fashion items, such as clothing. Turquoise is the natural complement of human complexion. As such, it flatters the appearance of the customer and therefore the products she purchases. Study the visualizations on Color Plate X.

As discussed in the following Chapter 18, the most "edible" colors for foods are in the peach and coral range. No other hues surpass them in appetite appeal.

However, for the *display* of foods, turquoise and blue for walls and fixtures are well prescribed. Meats look redder and more luscious. Packaged foods stand out conspicuously. And because blue is both universally liked and visually retiring, it is almost impossible to surpass.

Good color styling for stores involves variety, interest, and a constant change of pace. A riot of colors, however, should be avoided, for it may distract from the products on display. Nor should colors be picked "out of the air," so to speak. High individuality may run contrary to public taste, and overstyled decoration may defeat its own purpose.

Where colors are to be used at the point of sale and in relatively small areas, strong contrast should be considered. Light-colored merchandise can be featured against such deep hues as Maroon, Walnut Brown, Forest Green, Navy Blue. Here is a more specific suggestion: for wall color, Bright Yellow will hold maximum visibility. Eye attraction can be assured with a Fire Red or Vivid Orange sign. Trim fixtures or shelving should be in Sapphire Blue, Vivid Blue, or Navy Blue. Keep shelves white to provide sharp contrast with the packages or merchandise and to reflect light in normally shades areas. A combination like this is a "natural," because it has vital elements of compulsion, as well as emotional delight. No average person could miss it, and no one could say it was not in good taste.

With the more fashionable merchandise, other principles are to be followed and capitalized upon. The ideal background is not gray, but a toned color which strikes an average between white and black, and between color purity and neutral gray—all at one and the same time! Such muted colors as Rose, Pale Gold, Fern Green, Colonial Green, Smoky Blue will all give fair emphasis to white or light tints, as well as to pure, rich, and deep colors. While they lack impulse, they have a refinement that may be suitable for fashion products, or perhaps for beauty salons.

Again with respect to lighting, the eye will always concentrate on brightness rather than fight against dimness. If the general illumination is fluorescent, local incandescent light in spots or floods may be a necessary adjunct. It is one thing to be able to see clearly and another thing to find character, depth, plasticity, and texture in what is seen. Here is where store lighting differs from industrial. Textured products — furniture, carpeting, towels — need directional light for their rich beauty to be revealed. Shiny products — china, glassware, jewelry — similarly need sharp highlights and shadows. Without this, the merchandise may look "flat" and mediocre. If sharp highlights are wanted, black may be used as a local background, but should be surrounded by a more pleasing color such as blue to create eye appeal.

Lastly, for point of purchase areas, texture should not be neglected. Warm wood tones may be desirable in men's and women's fashions, shoes, and the like. Dull textures will complement shiny and glittery products. Lustrous textures will enhance soft goods. The eye is sensitive to texture, along with color. Variety being the spice of life, good designers will introduce novelty and work with all manner of things, from fish nets to sea shells, from brass lamps to glass globes, from driftwood to balloons — all to excite the sense and ring the bells of cash registers.

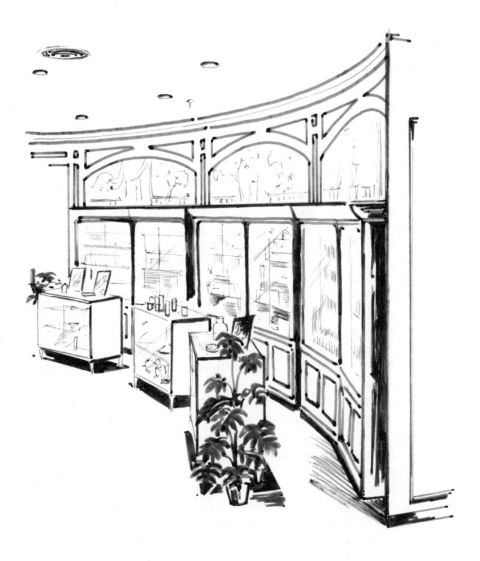

CHAPTER EIGHTEEN

Food Service

With foods, food display, and food service, color is inevitably involved throughout. First, the food itself displays myriad colors — the lush reds, mellow browns, the greens and yellows and orange tints of vegetables and fruits. Then, color is evident in the package or container in which it is featured, the store or market in which it is displayed, the restaurant or home in which it is served, the napery, china — even the carpets, walls, furniture.

There is a definite art of color in food. It is important to those who deal with food in any way, and to those who willingly or reluctantly consume it. What may not be properly appreciated is the fact that a sizable fund of research has been devoted to the matter of color and food, and much of it has direct and practical application.

It may seem a bit farfetched to speak of physiological responses to color in relationship to appetite, but perhaps not. One maker of chocolate candy found that sugar coating in a variety of hues (all with the same flavor) sold better than plain white or brown. Few customers know that butter — the expensive spread — is tinted for color control, just as is margarine. Butter that is too white may resemble lard, and butter that is too "goldenrod" may appear rancid. People demand the right shade (in countless other foodstuffs as well) and will accept or reject a product on its appearance — nutrition aside.

Basic to color and appetite perhaps are certain direct associations and certain known responses to the stimulation of color. Bright and warm colors (red, orange, yellow) tend to stimulate the autonomic nervous system of man — including digestion — while soft and cool colors tend to retard it. With birds and animals also, it has been found that reddish or yellowish light will excite hunger, while blue and green light discourage it.

In psychological studies of appetite appeal in color, a specific food palette is clearly revealed. Although not all persons will feel the same about colors or have the same reactions, by and large there are common denominators worthy of attention in the food industry.

To run through the hues of the spectrum, a peak in appetite appeal is found in the red-orange and orange region, where such hues seem to arouse the most agreeable sensations. There is a drop off at yellow-orange, and a pickup at yellow. Toward yellow-green, however, a low point is found. Although yellow-green may seem fashionable enough when applied to clothing or home furnishings, it is distasteful when applied to foods.

Pleasure is again restored in cool green and blue-green (turquoise), followed by another drop in purples.

Most readers will perhaps agree with these conclusions, psychological though they are. There is good appetite in tints such as Coral, Peach, Soft Yellow, Light Green, in richer colors such as Vermilion, Flamingo, Pumpkin, Bright Yellow. Blue-greens such as Aqua and Turquoise, while seldom associated with food itself, nonetheless are well regarded and well liked—and suggest an ideal foil or background for the display of food.

Poor colors are found in purplish reds, purple, violet, yellow-green, greenish yellow, orange yellow, gray, and most olive, "mustardy" tones, and grayed tones in general.

There are other fine points that sensitive mortals will express. Pink seems sweet. Candy colors suggest pastels. Wines are liked in pink, golden yellow, claret red.

The same appetite colors do not apply to all foods. Colored bread, once introduced, failed completely. Although "pretty" colors seem appropriate to cake frostings and cookies, they would be heartily rejected if used for mashed potatoes. A glass of purple grape juice would be relished — but not a purple gravy or consomme.

Colors for foods involve personal and emotional interpretations. No generalizations can be accepted as absolute. Nevertheless, it is good policy to avoid personal views for a more objective approach to the way in which most persons seem to react.

In food display cool blues such as Turquoise and Sapphire have been used quite successfully for backgrounds and fixtures in the sale of meat. White trays may be a necessary element here to suggest cleanliness. A food store at large could be Coral or Flamingo to inspire an active mood—offset perhaps by Peach, Yellow, Light Green, Pumpkin, or other appetite hues. That which the consumer sees ought to look "good enough to eat"; at least, there is good reason to apply such reasoning rather than disregard it and give in to personal hunches.

In food service — cocktail lounges, restaurants, cafeterias, coffee shops, snack bars — research has shown that the value of a color like Flamingo or Pumpkin for wall areas creates a generally active mood (see Color Plate XI). White, Vermilion, Turquoise, or Shapphire Blue can be used for accents. In one poll conducted in a cafeteria, a clean coral (peach) tone was voted the most appetizing of all. Turquoise blue was liked as a tile background to the steam tables.

In table accessories, cloths, dishes, the appetite palette is once again practical. A school cafeteria doubled the sale of salads by putting them on green plates. White, pink, aqua, pastel green, and yellow, by public confirmation, surpass other colors as being most desirable in food service. A decorator might dispute this with good right, but the conclusion is based on impersonal studies of average reactions. A southern restaurant, despite a good chef in the kitchen, had to repaint its dark purple walls. A French airline had to dispose of a chartreuse cabin after complaints of airsickness and nausea. Reflections from the bulkheads apparently made the passengers look sick and, therefore, feel sick.

Finally, there is the matter of illumination. In food service, warm light is almost imperative. The most savory meal would be rejected if served under mercury or sodium-vapor light. (This has been tested and proved.) One new principal in restaurants is to have a versatile lighting installation, in which a bright flood can be used for the noon hour rush and a soft diffusion of warmth for the evening dinner. In one instance the brilliance of the environment attracts the hungry man into the establishment and out in a hurry, whereas the homelike or candlelike atmosphere invites relaxation and repose — and a big check.

Food is big business. All too often it may lack a pleasing and friendly touch that color could help provide. Man has to eat. If he is at the mercy of this necessity, it would seem wise (and profitable) to offer his provender in a way that will delight his eye and charm his emotions, not merely cater to the pangs of his stomach.

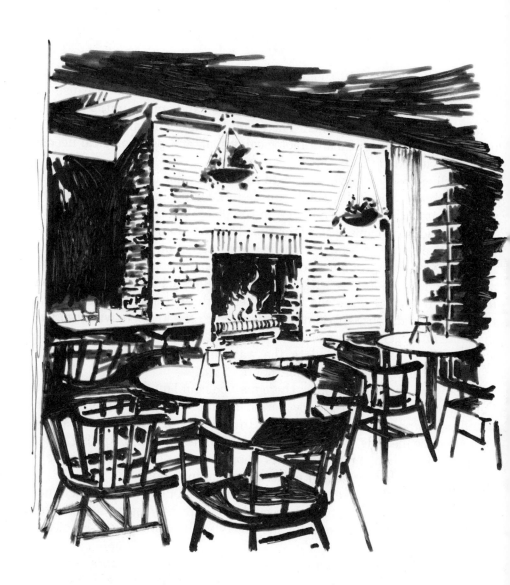

CHAPTER NINETEEN

Apartments and Homes

Mass housing, apartment complexes in all income groups, the concentration of people in retirement homes and convalescent homes because of extended life spans, all present great problems (and opportunities) to the architect and interior designer. There will be more and more need for a better understanding of man's biological, visual, and psychological needs, such as reviewed in this book.

Preceding chapters have dealt with the use of color in offices, industrial plants, schools, hospitals, motels and hotels, shops and stores, food service. Let attention now be directed to the places in which people *live*.

In a broad way man's leisure, the time he has to himself and to his family, has two main divisions — housing and recreation (see Color Plates XII and XIII). Housing may concern the specification of color for living areas, kitchens, bedrooms, bathrooms. In so-called luxury apartments, the living room may be large and the kitchen and dinette small, whereas in the low cost flat, most space may be devoted to the kitchen, with the living room no larger than is needed to hold a television set and a few chairs. These differences accommodate the ways in which people with much money and little money pass their hours.

In the mass housing complex there may be coin laundries, lobbies, perhaps a barber shop and beauty parlor, a drug store, boutique, tobacco stand, all in need of color treatment. In facilities devoted to recreation, there may be meeting rooms, parlors, game rooms, a library, bowling alley, woodworking shop, arts and crafts shop, courts devoted to handball, squash, tennis, basketball, an enclosed swimming pool.

Except for good light reflection in some instances, little of scientific functionalism necessarily has to be respected. Consequently, as in Color Plates XII and XIII, the choice of color can pretty well include any or all of the standards.

Assuming that a home is a man's—and/or woman's—castle where freedom should reign, the emotional delights of the occupation should by all means be catered to and gratified. Taste here should be personal.

Books on interior decoration exist by the score. Many of them are excellent and offer splendid guidance in room layout, furniture arrangement, and color harmony. However, to this writer the decoration of homes is and should be a personal affair. Despite many years of experience in the *functional* specifications of color for commercial and institutional interiors, the author is ever reluctant to offer advice regarding a home. It is often much easier to do five or six floors of general business space than to settle the details of a private office. People will utilize reason when devoting attention to the needs of others, but they will resent personal intrusions on their own conceptions of taste.

This is as it should be — but not always is. Most human beings have deep feelings about color. Their attitude towards it may be like their religious or political convictions — not to be disturbed without a strong emotional response. No color scheme to the knowledge of this writer, no interior, holds universal appeal. Tradition may seem archaic to a modern, and modernism may seem ludicrous to a fancier of period styles. As for color itself, differences of view are even more pronounced. Almost every hue has its "lovers" and "haters." And when one person uses what another person dislikes, this second mortal may secretly or openly wonder at the wretched taste of the first.

There could be a "scientific" way of decorating a home, but very few would like it. For example, the living room could, with good cause, be a medium tone of rose to create a soft, warm, and cheerful atmosphere. The dining room could have peach walls and turquoise blue furnishings to inspire appetites. The kitchen could be in yellow with red and blue accents to establish a lively effect and make time pass swiftly. The bedroom could be in pink or aqua like spring itself. But who would care? Logic does not usually prevail where color and human personality are involved.

It seems important for a person to obtain his own way with color. Advice can be accepted in matters of design, form, arrangement — or even in the particular tone of a color for a particular setting. But *the color itself* ought to spring from the heart. If it does not, the home owner may well end up dissatisfied, if not distraught and unhappy.

Some years ago, the author conceived the word *psychodecor*. He has written one book and numerous articles on the psychological and psychiatric aspects of color. In the process he has learned much about the subtle peculiarities of the human psyche.

For example, and in a broad sense, people may be classified as extroverts and introverts. The terms are those of Carl Jung. The extroverts by nature are outgoing and take delight in bright and warm colors. The introverts, on the other hand, are more introspective and likely to prefer subdued and cool colors. In a similar way, it is natural for extroverts to like innovation and modernism in furniture, while the introvert, needing reason to support his taste, may prefer the sentiment and historic dignity attached to that which is traditional. Certainly, no one is right or wrong here, for no amount of debate could settle anything.

A person hazards much in venturing to give advice on color. A timid woman might be told to use bright colors and get over her moody ways. Yet bright colors could well make this person so extremely self-conscious that she might become even more timid and lugubrious. The excitable woman, advised to surround herself with soft and subdued hues, may find that such an environment "bottles up" the spirit and makes a person all the more nervous. Incidentally, these facts are known in the field of psychiatry, and principles based on them are used in the decoration of elementary schools, and general and mental hospitals.

So it is poor wisdom to let the individuality of others impose on your own taste for color. There is a deep and profound satisfaction in color that is well worth the emotional effort of bringing it forth. Architects and interior decorators should consider it part of their trade to "psychoanalyze" their clients (the good ones do). Color can make people happy — and unhappy. Where attention is given to human predilections, to a skillful and talented interpretation of the heart-felt desires of others, decoration becomes a high art. It is inspired to great originality and variety, for it acquires shades of expression as diverse as those that compose human character.

If advice is to be given, let it present the facts, phenomena, and case history experiences which affect the use of any and all color. Here are a few notes and observations. Colors will seem more intense in large areas than in small. The color of a paint chip or on a color card will not appear the same on a wall.

Be particularly careful of pale luminous colors like yellow. They are most deceptive in a chip. On the walls of a room, and because of high reflectance, the light colors will "bounce" back and forth and hence increase in purity. For example, if a cheerful yellow (or chartreuse, peach, or pink) is wanted, choose the chip and then dilute the paint with as much as fifty percent white — the color on the chip and that on the wall will then probably look the same.

Don't fear pure colors, such as vermilion red. While they may not stand full daylight, in a normal interior with draperies, blinds, and artificial light, they will soften down. If you really like color, do not deprive yourself. If four walls are too many, put the brilliant color on one and a neutral on the others.

If deep colors are preferred, use similar precautions and keep in mind the principle described in Chapter 10 on color value. In an artificially lit room the dark color can stand some reflected light. During the day it will be perfectly all right. However, be cautious about dark colors (or brilliant ones) on ceilings. They may crowd down in a disturbing way.

Above all, for a home, have the courage of your convictions and feelings. Color is one of the natural delights of this world. It is the rule of nature, not the exception, and much of the good life resides in it.

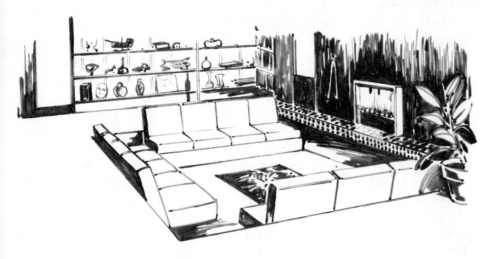

CHAPTER TWENTY

Practical Color Organization

The American Institute of Architects is a member of the Inter-Society Color Council, an organization devoted to technical and general problems of color. A committee on the presentation of colored building products has been set up to find practical ways in which manufacturers of building materials can make effective color presentations and to resolve questions of standardization, identification, and uniformity.

There are a number of complex instruments—colorimeters, spectrophotometers—available to measure color in scientific terms. They are designed for manufacturers' use rather than for architects. What may concern the architect are physical standards—color systems of swatches or chips and simple methods of color description, notation, naming, and reference.

Architectural color standards have not been successfully established or adopted in the United States. British architects, however, have set up Colour Range BS2660, which establishes 101 basic colors as standards. Major English manufacturers of paint and other products such as ceramic tile make these colors available. A progressive manufacturer of products for the building industry may offer additional colors for the sake of individuality and competitive advantage.

American industry tends to resist color standardization as too limiting and too discouraging of creative color styling, although Federal Standard 595 defines the colors used by most branches of the Government. It consists of over 400 mounted chips with code numbers. The colors of many products purchased by the Government meet these specifications.

The Germans have a similar standard, DIN-Farbenkarte. The Japan Color Research Institute has likewise set standards known as Chroma Cosmos 5000, which is discussed below. A fairly new and beautiful system of color standards has been issued by the Scandinavian Color Institute of Stockholm, Sweden. It is known as the Natural Color System and is described as being based "completely on man's natural perception of color." About 1500 colors have been released in various forms (atlas, color blocks, fans, and cards).

Standardizing agencies here and abroad cover many products too numerous to mention here: the American National Standards Institute, the British Standards Institution, Japanese Industrial Standards; there are similar organizations in other nations. (A checklist by Birren, "Color Identification and Nomenclature: a History," has been published in *Color Research and Application*, Vol. 4, No. 1, Spring, 1979.)

One of the most beautiful and elaborate color systems ever developed is that of the Japanese Color Research Institute, Chroma Cosmos 5000. Issued in 1978, it contains 5000 individually coated and mounted chips, beautifully featured on 23 double charts (10¼ x 29 inches) with an

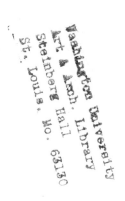

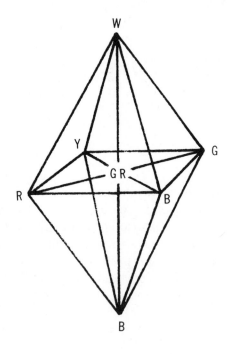

Color Pyramid, A. Hofler, 1897.

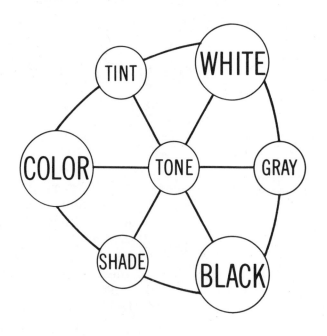

Color Triangle.

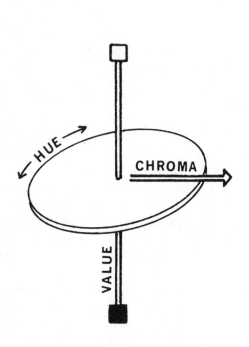

Order of major color dimensions.

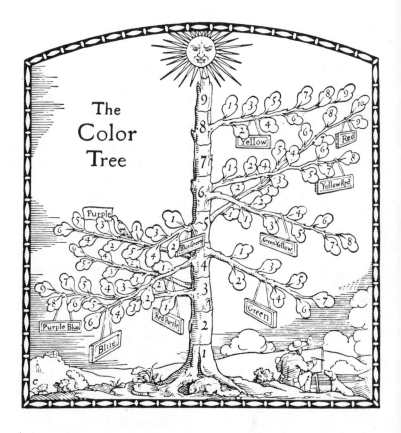

Romantic concept of Munsell Color Tree by T. M. Cleland.

additional folder of introduction and explanation. The entire presentation is organized according to the Munsell System and the ISCC-NBS Method of Designating Colors (to be described). While its cost is considerable ($1,500) it is essential for anyone who would like to have firm control of the eternal problem of color identification.

Visual color organization is easily expressed in graphics. A widely recognized chart or graph is that of A. Höfler; it dates to 1897 and has been referred to in many books on psychology over the years. It consists of a double pyramid. At the top apex is the color white; at the bottom, black; between them a scale of neutral grays. On the four corners of the central connecting base are red, yellow, green, and blue, the four primaries universally accepted in the field of vision. (The physicist identifies red, green, and blue-violet primaries, while the artist and process printer use magenta, yellow, and cyan blue.) All colors seen by the eye lie within the outer boundaries of the Höfler pyramid. This type of schematic concept was followed by other authorities: the American Ogden Rood and the German Wilhelm Ostwald developed a double cone rather than a double pyramid; Albert H. Munsell visualized a sphere or "tree."

In simple terminology, pure colors, which run about the circumference of a color solid, are termed *hues*. The colors that progress from lightness to darkness are known as *values*. The colors that run from neutral gray toward pure hues are characterized by *chroma* or saturation. A simple color triangle plots color variations with respect to pure hue, white, and black; and tint, tone, shade, and gray. All these variations fit within the Höfler pyramid and most color solids devised in the past.

A large part of the world of color recognizes the principles of color identification set forth by Albert H. Munsell as early as 1898 but since improved upon by leading and dedicated experts both here and abroad. Today the Munsell System is the most widely used method of color notation in existence. Knowledge of it is recommended to architects and interior designers, as well as to anyone else confronted by the problem of color designation.

A charming sketch of the Munsell color tree is shown in this chapter. It was done by T. M. Cleland, a graphic artist, in 1921. A Cleland design of the Munsell color circle is also shown, as is a more sober view of the Munsell solid. The system follows the general shape of a sphere, somewhat bulbous in parts. Because pure colors do not have equal value, hues such as yellow are placed near the white apex, and hues such as blue near the black apex. Again, colors with strong chroma or saturation, such as vivid red, extend farther from the neutral-gray axis than do weak colors such as blue-green. There are 10 major hues: red, yellow-red (orange), yellow, green-yellow, green, blue-green, blue, purple-blue, purple, and red-purple. They are further divided into 100 subhues. There are 9 value stages (vertical) from ideal white to black. Chroma or saturation stages (horizontal) vary according to the purity of the key hue.

Hue is denoted by a symbolic letter (sometimes preceded by a number to correspond to its location on the 100-step equation). Value is denoted by a number from 1 to 9 (or in between). Chroma is also denoted by a number indicating degree of departure from the neutral-gray axis. A brilliant primary red, for example, might be indicated by 5R 4/14 (4 value, 14 chroma). A high-value, moderate-chroma pink might be 5R 8/4; a low-value, medium-chroma maroon, 5R 2/6; a medium-value, weak-chroma rose, 5R 5/2.

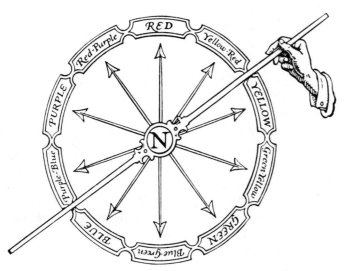

Cleland's drawing of Munsell Color Circle.

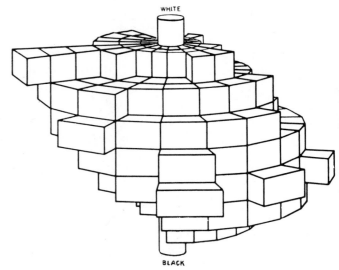

The Munsell Color Solid.

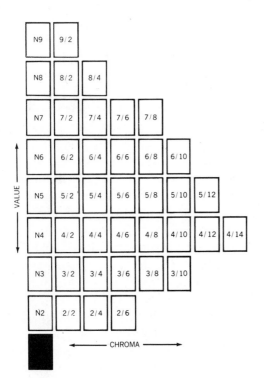

Munsell Notations for the color Red.

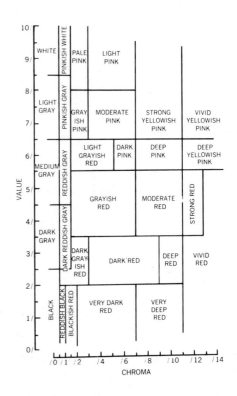

ISCC-NBS designations for the color Red.

A complete Munsell System, with glossy-finish chips, includes over 1,500 colors. The Japanese Chroma Cosmos 5000 system in the same way identifies 5000 chips! Color standards can thus be readily notated with a few letters and numbers. Scientists have measured all Munsell notations and given them technical identification in what are known as CIE XYZ terms.

In 1955 the National Bureau of Standards (Department of Commerce) issued a remarkable work: *The Inter-Society Color Council–National Bureau of Standards* (ISCC–NBS) *Method of Designating Colors and A Dictionary of Color Names*. It resulted from a series of conferences sponsored by the ISCC and was ably prepared by Deane B. Judd and Kenneth L. Kelly of the Bureau. Based largely on the Munsell Color System (which had been scientifically renotated by a group of experts), it developed a language of color using everyday English words to describe blocks that corresponded to sections of individual Munsell charts.

In the two diagrams shown one gives color notations (numbers) for a Munsell basic red, 5R; the other gives descriptive names for the same colors. The four Munsell notations previously referred to translate into the ISCC–NBS method as follows:

5R 4/14, strong red
5R 8/4, moderate pink
5R 2/6, very dark red
5R 5/2, grayish red

The 1955 publication gives color names to 31 key Munsell charts. There are 267 blocks devoted to the charts, each block containing descriptive terms.

The descriptive terms within the 267 blocks are further used to describe colors included in other systems and collections: Federal Standard 595, the Maerz and Paul Dictionary of Color, the Plochere Color System, the Horticultural Colour Charts, the Descriptive Color Names Dictionary of the (Ostwald) Color Harmony Manual, the Standard Color Card of America of the Textile Color Card Association, and others. In effect, all the colors *named* in these collections are identified by the ISCC–NBS method. Over 10,000 names from the above collections are alphabetically arranged. Anyone looking for a comprehensive list of color names will find them here—and be able to approximate their visual appearance in Munsell colors!

A further refinement of the ISCC–NBS Method has recently been introduced. In 1965 what are known as Centroid Color Charts were produced, thanks to much effort by Kenneth L. Kelly. There are 18 charts, which contain 267 mounted chips. These chips are directly related to the 267 blocks mentioned above and have been given numbers from 1 to 267. The blocks are plotted against the charts of the Munsell System.

To identify a specimen of paint, textile, plastic, or paper, follow these steps.

1. Find it definitely or approximately in the Munsell Book of Color. Give the color a Munsell designation, or interpolate it if it lies between Munsell chips.

2. Refer to the Color Names Dictionary. The Munsell designation is described on the equivalent Munsell black-and-white chart.

3. If you would like to know what other names or terms have been used for the color, look it up in the Synonymous list of the Color Names Dictionary. For example, 5R 4/14, described as strong red above, is found

on block #12 on the Centroid Charts, which lists 93 names; 5R 8/4, described as moderate pink, on block #5, 62 names; 5R 2/6, described as very dark red, on block #17, 15 names; 5R 5/2, described as grayish red, on block #19, 158 names!

4. If you want a general idea of the color's appearance, refer to its number (1 to 267) on the Centroid Charts.

For scientific and technical data on color identification and measurement the following references are suggested: Method of Specifying Color by the Munsell System, ANSI/ASTM D1535–68 [Z138.5] and Practice for Spectrophotometry and Description of Color in CIE 1931 System [Z138.2], available from American National Standards Institute, 1430 Broadway, New York, N.Y. 10018; Chroma Cosmos 5000, from Japan Color Research Institute, 1–19, Nishiazabu 3-chome, Minato-Ku, Tokyo 106, Japan; Munsell Book of Color, Glossy Finish Collection, from Munsell Color, 2441 North Calvert Street, Baltimore, MD 21218; Color: Universal Language and Dictionary of Names, from U.S. Government Printing Office, Washington, D.C. 20402, SD Catalog No. C13.10:440; ISCC–NBS Centroid Color Charts, Standard Sample No. 2106, from Office of Standard Reference Materials, National Bureau of Standards, Washington, D.C. 20234.

APPENDIX A

The Historical Background

Anyone who works with color in architecture and interior design should appreciate the ancient and fascinating heritage that lies behind the art. This appendix and the one to follow will tell this story with two purposes in mind. The first is to identify color with virtually all aspects of human culture, past and present, and the second to present authentic data on period styles and traditions for those who may, in these times, wish to echo and resurrect the beauty of the past. This author has devoted much time to the historical background of color. Two of his books have dealt at length with it: *Color, a Survey in Words and Pictures*; *Color for Interiors*. Both are recommended, and both have been substantially referred to in the preparation of the two appendixes herewith.

To begin at the beginning, the beauty of Egyptian, Chaldean, Greek, and Oriental art arose not out of esthetics alone but out of religion and superstition. Here is where civilization was founded and formed. Art was functional and practical in that it was symbolic. The Egyptians used it to "deny the physical evidence of death." The *ziggurats* of Babylon were veritable charts of mysticism in architecture. The palaces of China were painstakingly designed to emblem the five elements, the two essences, and the ultimate principle of the universe. The early sculpture of Greece was not abstract in conception but was used to personify gods and mortals.

The evidence of history pretty well defeats the attempt to speak of creative art in the modern sense. Why was the palette always simple: red, yellow, gold, green, blue, purple, pink, white, black? How could the Greek mind, so sensitive to form, to balance and the harmony of line and mass, make so little effort to be subtle with hue? Beechey very aptly remarks of Greek architectural decoration: "We observe that the practice we allude to does not appear . . . to be the result of any occasional caprice or fancy, but of a generally established system; for the colors of the several parts do not seem to have materially varied in any two instances with which we are acquainted . . . We can scarcely doubt that one particular color was appropriated by general consent or practice to each of the several parts of the buildings."

If the Greeks or any civilized men before them were trying to express highly personal feelings, how may one account for this apparently matter-of-fact and commonplace use of the spectrum? The answer must be that the ancient artist had definite reasons for color, just as he had sound ideas about architecture. He was a humble votary who gave himself not to the whims of his own individuality but to the social and religious consciousness of his people. He was not a creator in the modern sense but an interpreter. He did not seek to inspire men with *his* sense of beauty, but to follow dictates and principles set before him by others.

When one realizes that practically every surviving archaeological record of ancient times is a temple or tomb — not an office building, state capitol, library, museum, school, or home — one may appreciate that religious thought and expression ruled the day.

In religion, man included his philosophy and science. The great principles of nature and the vital forces of the universe were personified by gods and goddesses. Religion held sway not only over the spirit of man (as today) but also over his mind and every institution of government. The foremost brains of antiquity — teachers, scientists, philosophers, priests, physicians — were the mystics. They guided the empire, regulated the affairs of war and peace, commerce and industry, and formed the intelligence and culture of nations.

The sun was the principle of good, master of sky and earth, sustaining all life and controlling the universe. To the Egyptian it was Osiris. To the Persian it was Mithras. To the Hindu it was Brahma. To the Chaldean it was Bel. To the Greek it was Adonis and Apollo. God was the supreme deity associated with light. His emanations gave hue to the rainbow. They pervaded all space, put breath and spirit into the body of man. The golden ornaments of priests and the crowns of kings referred to the sun. Red, yellow, green, blue, purple were a part of these emanations, each significant, each emblematic of divine forces.

In Egypt yellow and gold were tokens of the sun. The color of man was red. Green represented the eternity of nature. Purple was the hue of earth. Blue, like the heavens, was sacred to justice. It was worn on the breastplates of Egyptian priests to indicate the holiness of their judgments.

Osiris, the father of the Egyptian trinity, was green. His son Horus was white. Set, the deity of evil, was black. Shu, who separated earth from sky, was red.

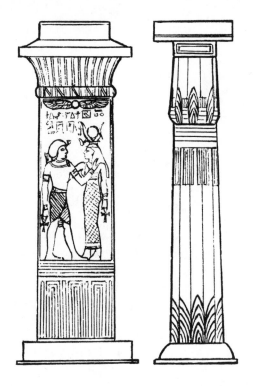

Columns of Karnak, Luxor, Egypt, 1400 B.C.

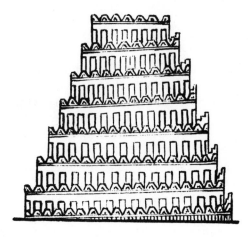

Temple of Nebuchadnezzar, Babylon, 500 B.C.

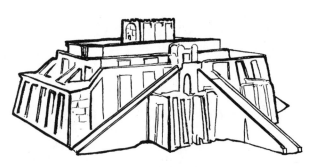

Mountain of God, Ur, 2500 B.C.

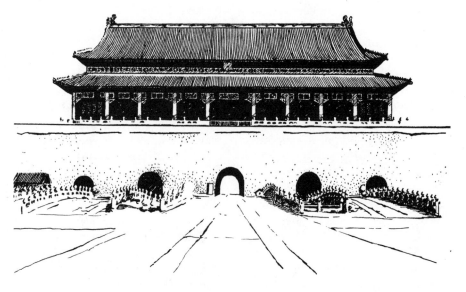

Chinese temple, Peking.

Amen, the god of life and reproduction, was blue.

Time was addressed as the "everlasting green one." The races of man were four in number — red for the Egyptians, yellow for the Asiatics, white for the peoples of the north, black for the Negro. In the ritualism of death, amulets and colors buried in the tomb of the deceased brought security until the time of resurrection. A green stone performed "the opening of the mouth," restoring speech to the corpse. The red *Tjet* gave the virtue of the blood of Isis. The red *Ab*, or heart amulet, preserved the soul of the physical body. The golden *Udjat* afforded health and protection. The red *Nefer* brought happiness and fortune. the brownish *Sma* caused breath to return.

All these involved significant works of art that glisten today in the glass cases of museums. Men in the time of Egypt were obviously not catering to vanity alone nor indulging themselves in mere artistic expression. Egyptian amulets, vignettes, coffin decorations, the rubrics of manuscripts, temples, sculptural ornaments, painting — all had purposes. They were designed to symbolize the Mysteries, to invoke the favor of the gods, to seek victory over nature, affliction, plague, drought, and death, to serve life first, last, and always. Where the modern artist speaks of the intrinsic beauty of color and its ability to thrill the emotions through the eye, the Egyptian was primarily concerned with a language of color that was precise rather than vague in its meaning.

In the Orient this same use of color prevailed. Gods were identified by hues. In India Brahma was yellow; Siva the destroyer was black. Yellow was likewise sacred to Buddha and to Confucius. Green was sacred to Mohammed and is still worn in the turban of the Moslem who has made a pilgrimage to Mecca.

Architecturally, however, most color symbolism came from the study of astrology. This science originated in Chaldee and was practiced two thousand years before the birth of Christ. Great temples were dedicated to the gods of the heavens and designated in color to symbolize the seven planets.

Throughout Asia color, architecture, and design answered to the Mysteries. Everything had meaning. Art was created out of belief. There were few abstractions as today, murals that attempt to spiritualize commerce, progress, and whatnot through the emotional implications of hue. The Oriental had a story to tell, and his symbols and hues were as fixed in his mind as the letters of the alphabet.

In Mongolia the earth was conceived as being a high mountain called Sumur. "In the beginning was only water and a frog, which gazed into the water. God turned this animal over and created the world on its belly. On each foot he built a continent, but on the naval of the frog he founded the Sumur Mountain. On the summit of this mountain is the North Star." The four sides of the mountain were hued. To the north was yellow. To the south was blue. To the east was white. To the west was red.

In China color was (and still is) inextricably woven into the culture of the race. Again the points of the compass were identified — black for the north, red for the south, green for the east, white for the west. (This association of color with the four quarters of the world has also been found in the culture of ancient Ireland and the Indians of North America.)

To the Chinese the primary colors were five in number, red, yellow, black, white, green (and blue). These hues were related to the five Chinese elements, fire, metal, wood, earth, and water, to the five happinesses, the five virtues, the five vices, the five precepts of faith.

Dynasties were known by hues, brown for the Sung Dynasty, green for the Ming, yellow for the Ch'ing. The emperor wore blue when he worshipped the sky, yellow when he worshipped the earth. He signed all edicts with vermilion ink. His officials wore colored buttons atop their caps to distinguish their rank. His grandchildren rode in purple sedans, his higher officials in blue, his lower officials in green.

In the Chinese theater the sacred person was indicated by a red face; the face of the boor was black, the villain white. These colors were as unmistakably clear in meaning as the black mustaches and blond curls of performers in a Victorian melodrama. They were understood by all, serf and king. To bless the emperor the priest chanted: "These white jewels are a prognostic of the great august white hairs to which your Majesty will reach. The red jewels are the august, healthful, ruddy countenance, and the green jewels are the harmonious fitness which your Majesty will establish far and wide."

Jewels and colors have always marked paradise and utopia. In the Hindu *Ramayana* the "other world" is described as follows:

The land is watered by lakes with golden lotuses. There are rivers by thousands, full of leaves of the color of sapphire and lapis lazuli; and the lakes, resplendent like the morning sun, are adorned by golden beds of red lotus. The country all around is covered by jewels and precious stones, with gay beds of blue lotus, golden-petalled. Instead of sand, pearls, gems, and gold form the banks of the rivers, which are overhung with trees of fire-bright gold. These trees perpetually bear flowers and fruit, give forth a sweet fragrance and abound with birds.

Similar descriptions, involving gems and colors, are found in the culture of the Buddhists, Japanese, Celts, Teutons, and the Incas and Aztecs of America. And biblical references are several.

Chinese, Hindu, Chaldean, and Egyptian learning was the basis of Greek and Roman culture. Naturally the color traditions of these earlier civilizations crossed the Hellespont to dwell on the continent north of the

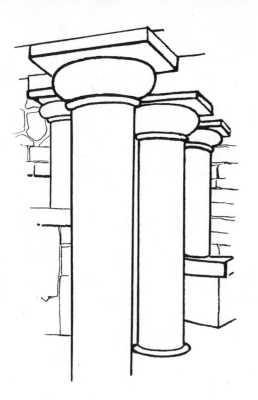

Greek frieze.

Columns, Palace of Minos, Knossos, Crete, 1500 B.C.

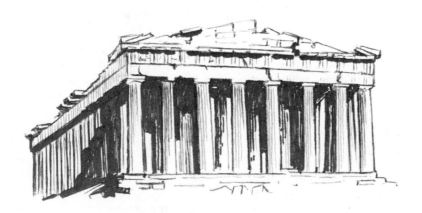

The Parthenon, 400 B.C.

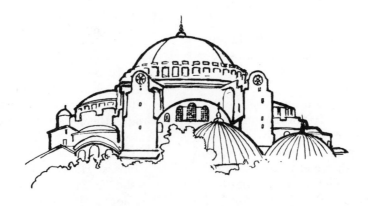

Hagia Sophia, Istanbul, 535 A.D.

Mediterranean. The old gods were given new names. Athena, wise in the arts of peace and war, was adorned with a yellow robe. Red was sacred to Ceres and to Dionysus. Pythagoras wrote of the two virgins of the temple, one veiled in a white robe, the other bedecked with the jewels of earthly treasures. A white robe symbolized purity, a red robe sacrifice and love, a blue robe altruism and integrity. When acting the Odyssey, the ancients wore purple to symbolize the sea wanderings of Odysseus. For the Iliad they wore scarlet in reference to the bloody battles of the poem.

Later in Rome purple became the imperial color, Caesar wearing it to personify Jupiter.

"Heaven is always a place of gems," wrote Aldous Huxley, and to this should be added color. Socrates in the *Phaedo* said: "In this other earth the colors are much purer and much more brilliant than they are down here. . . . The very mountains, the very stones have a richer gloss, a lovelier transparency and intensity of hue. The precious stones of this lower world, our highly prized carnelians, jaspers, emeralds and all the rest, are but the tiny fragments of these stones above. In the other earth there is no stone but is precious and exceeds in beauty every gem of ours."

Sculpture in Greece comprised the fashioning of effigies, gods and goddesses who lived and breathed and even vanished from one place to appear in another. One writer describes a freshly unearthed pediment: "Flesh, reddish in tone; globe of eyes yellow, iris green, with a hole in the center filled with black; black outlines to eyebrows and eyelids; hair and beard bright blue at the time of excavation, which disintegrated later to a greenish tone; circle of brown around the nipples."

But the color art of Greece has not been well preserved because of deterioration. Much of it was lost for centuries, during which artists and architects devoted themselves to the adoration of form and gave rebirth to classic styles in which color was sadly missing. Greek artists, however, gave symbolism to color just as did the savants of former times. Mythology told of the four ages of man, gold, silver, copper, and iron. The science of the universe as comprised of four elements, earth, fire, water, and air, led to the theory of Pythagoras that earth particles were cubical, fire particles tetrahedral, water particles icosahedral, air particles octahedral. The fifth solid, a dodecahedron, symbolized the ether. The sphere, perfect among all symmetrical solids, was reserved for the deity.

And once again colors were significantly applied, blue to symbolize earth, red for fire, green for water, and yellow for air. (Other designations were given later. Josephus in the first century spoke of white earth, red fire, purple water, blue air. Da Vinci in the fifteenth century related yellow to earth, red to fire, green to water, and blue to air.) Man himself was composed of colors and elements, his flesh and bone of blueness and earth, his bodily heat of redness and fire, his blood and fluids of greenness and water, the gases within him of yellowness and air.

One may trace the same august respect for color among other races throughout the world. The Druids of England used green, blue, and white in their rituals. In some civilizations human beings were sacrificed in a red temple draped with red hangings. The elements were controlled through incantations and rites that involved colors. The ceremonies of birth, circumcision, puberty, marriage, death were rich in color associations. Amulets, charms, and hues brought protection over the household, thwarted the evil eye, drove away disease.

As paganism died in Western countries, to be replaced by Christianity, color began to lose its importance. Yet not entirely. Cabalism spoke of a trinity of blue, yellow, and red. The Egyptian trinity of Osiris, Isis, and Horus, the Hindu trinity of Brahma, Vishnu, and Siva, the philosophic notion of life, birth, and death, of past, present, and future, of dawn, day, and dusk, gave way to a new theology. Now there was God the Father, Creator of the World, whose hue was blue to symbolize heaven and the spirit of man. God the Son was radiant in the fullness of day; His hue was yellow, the symbol of earth and the mind of man. God the Holy Ghost was the setting sun; His hue was red, the symbol of hell and the body of man.

The mystic struggled to preserve color traditions. He pointed to numerous references in the Bible, visions of the Lord, laws for the construction of the Tabernacle. The Tablets of the Law given to Moses had been fashioned of divine sapphire. A red carbuncle had shone from the prow of Noah's Ark. The Holy Grail had been green. In the Old Testament, Ezekiel gave several references to gems and colors. As for the Almighty, "And above the fermament that was over their heads was the likeness of a throne, as the appearance of a sapphire stone: and upon the likeness of the throne was the likeness as the appearance of a man above it." As for the heavenly environment, "Thou hast been in Eden the garden of God: every precious stone was thy covering, the sardius, topaz, and the diamond, the beryl, the onyx, and the jasper, the sapphire, the emerald, and the carbuncle, and gold."

In the New Testament, St. John the Divine had spoken of the New Jerusalem and its twelve foundations garnished with twelve different hues and jewels. He describes the great ethereal city as follows:

And the building of the wall of it was of jasper: and the city was pure gold, like unto clear glass.

And the foundations of the wall of the city were garnished with all manner of precious stones. The first foun-

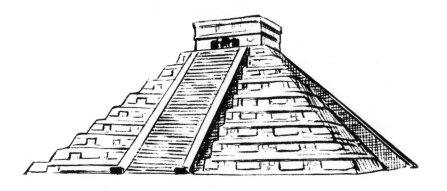

Pyramid of the Mayas, Mexico, 800 A.D.

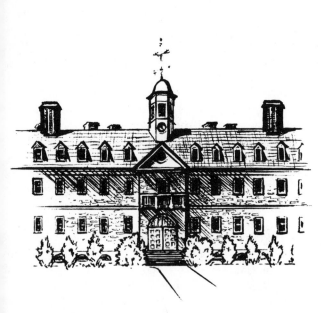

College of William and Mary, Williamsburg, Virginia, Christopher Wren.

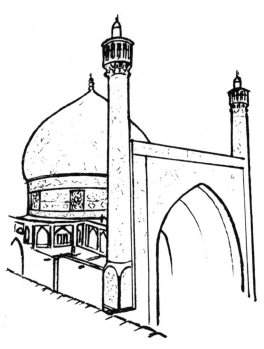

Imperial Mosque, Isfahan, Iran, 1500 A.D.

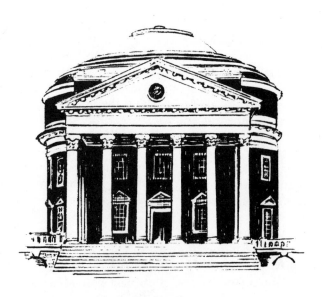

Rotunda, University of Virginia, Thomas Jefferson.

dation was jasper; the second, sapphire; the third, a chalcedony; the fourth, an emerald.

The fifth, sardonyx; the sixth, sardius; the seventh, chrysolyte; the eighth, beryl; the ninth, a topaz; the tenth, a chrysoprasus; the eleventh, a jacinth; the twelfth, an amethyst.

And the twelve gates were twelve pearls: every several gate was of one pearl: and the street of the city was pure gold, as it were transparent glass.

There was thought to be symbolism in all this, a key to the mysteries of life. But the Church turned from paganism, and the mystic was vanquished.

Yet his fervor did not pass entirely. It was revived by the alchemist and in medieval times glowed once more — black, the darkness and beginning of all things; white, the light of creation; red and gold, the glory of the sun. Alchemy influenced the early Gothic architect, and like the craftsman of old he used color to symbolic purpose. But his iniquity was discovered and his works covered with whitewash. In 1652 one Elias Ashmole wrote of such an event — the destruction of an alchemical design in color on an arched wall in Westminster Abbey. "Nothwithstanding it has pleased some, to wash the *Originall* over with a *Plasterer's* whited Brush." . . .

With the reader's permission, let the story now be retold with as many specific references as possible. As has been stated, and except for a few notable survivals, not much remains of color in ancient *exterior* architectural adornment, and even less of *interior*. Yet it is true that a Classical (symbolic) tradition for color prevailed more or less up to the time of the Renaissance. Colors were not intuitively or impulsively used, but were used with strict respect for the Mysteries.

To go back again, Egyptian color in architecture and decoration was simple, the red hue of man, the purple of earth, the yellow of the sun, the green of nature, the blue of divine truth. There still are vestiges of red pigment on the face of the Sphinx. The chambers of the Great Pyramid, however, far older, are faded and indicate but an elemental symbolism. Generally the ceilings of tombs and temples were blue and embellished with pictures of the constellations. The floors were green and blue like the meadows of the Nile. The brilliant color at Karnak (seen in person by this writer) featured the same red, yellow, green, blue that was part of the Egyptian Mysteries. Limestone, sandstone, granite, flinty diorite, the materials of the time, were glazed and painted to conform to the dictates of religion. The king wore a high white crown to symbolize his dominion over upper Egypt, and his treasury here was called the "White House." A flat red crown proclaimed his mastery over lower Egypt and the treasury of the "Red House."

In the beautifully preserved tomb of Sennefer at Thebes, dating back 3,400 years (also visited in person) great decorations, in bold colors, cover the walls and vaulted ceiling. All is symbolic, both as to hue and design motifs, for the tomb contains portraits of Sennefer's wives, children, domestic servants, dancers, plus ornate hieroglyphics and the furnishings, equipments, foods and wines necessary to Egyptian life at the time. The flesh of men was portrayed as a rich terra cotta red, that of women as a golden ocher. Otherwise, there was white, yellow, green, blue, black.

As in Egypt, so Mesopotamia and Asia also used color. Here the study of astrology led to a symbolism for color that dominated all architecture. C. Leonard Woolley in a joint expedition of the British Museum and the Museum of Pennsylvania unearthed the ancient *ziggurat*, the "Mountain of God," at Ur between Bagdad and the Persian Gulf, one of the oldest buildings in the world.

The tower measured about 200 feet in length, 150 feet in width, and was originally about 70 feet high. It was built in four stages, a great solid mass of brickwork. At the top was the square shrine of Nannar, the Moon-God. Woolley found an absence of straight lines. Horizontal planes bulged outward, vertical planes were slightly convex — a subtlety once thought to be of Greek origin and quite evident in the Parthenon.

The lowest stage of this tower was black, the uppermost red. The shrine was covered with blue glazed tile, the roof with gilded metal. Woolley wrote, "These colors had their mystical significance and stood for the various divisions of the universe, the dark underworld, the habitable earth, the heavens and the sun."

More pretentious *ziggurats* have been unearthed. In the fifth century B.C., Herodotus wrote of Ecbatana:

The Medes built the city now called Ecbatana, the walls of which are of great size and strength, rising in circles one within the other. The plan of the place is, that each of the walls should out-top the one beyond it by the battlements. The nature of the ground, which is a gentle hill, favors this arrangement in some degree, but it was mainly effected by art. The number of the circles is seven, the royal palace and the treasuries standing within the last. The circuit of the outer wall is very nearly the same with that of Athens. Of this wall the battlements are white, of the next black, of the third scarlet, of the fourth blue, of the fifth orange; all these are colored with paint. The two last have their battlements coated respectively with silver and gold. All these fortifications Deioces had caused to be raised for himself and his own palace.

Herodotus to all indications referred to the great temple of Nebuchadnezzar at Barsippa, the Birs Nimroud. Uncovered in modern times, its bricks bear the stamp of the Babylonian monarch who apparently rebuilt it in the seventh century B.C. It was 272 feet square at its base and rose in seven stages, each stage being set back away from a central point. Of this building James Fergusson wrote:

This temple, as we know from the decipherment of the cylinders which were found on its angles, was dedicated to the seven planets of heavenly spheres, and we find it consequently adorned with the colors of each. The lower, which was also richly paneled, was black, the color of Saturn; the next, orange, the color of Jupiter; the third, red, emblematic of Mars; the fourth, yellow, belonging to the sun; the fifth and sixth, green and blue respectively, as dedicated to Venus and Mercury, and the upper probably white, that being the color belonging to the moon, whose place in the Chaldean system would be uppermost.

To digress for a moment, in China similar conventions were followed. In the humble dwelling, homes of more than two stories were avoided. In his *Outlines of Chinese Symbolism*, C. A. S. Williams writes:

Height is also limited by the belief that good spirits soar through the air at a height of 100 feet, a restriction of moment only in great temples and other buildings on city walls. Climate and the belief that good spirits blow from the south have decided the orientation of buildings with a southern aspect and windowless north walls. The abhorrence of a tortuous path, which is a characteristic of evil spirits, has given us the spirit walls which define so many gateways. For the same reason we have the up-curved roof edge with its dragon finials.

When a home was built, red firecrackers were exploded from the upper beam of the roof. A piece of red cloth was suspended to promote felicity. Green pine branches were placed atop the scaffolding to deceive wandering evil spirits and lead them to believe they were passing over a forest.

In the palaces and temples of China one finds color symbolism everywhere. As in the Forbidden City of Peking the hues emblem the five elements, virtues, vices, etc. Red shows as the positive essence, the heavenly and masculine principle. Yellow shows as the negative essence, the earthly and feminine principle. Thus the walls of Peking are red, symbolic of the south, the sun, happiness. The roofs are yellow, symbolic of the earth.

Let this story now lead into Greece, Rome, and into the Renaissance, and then through Europe into France, and England.

In the palace of Minos at Knossos in Crete, unearthed by Arthur Evans and dating back to 1600 B.C. and before, are restorations that are quite vivid in color. There were wall paintings in red oxide, golden ocher, blue, brown, black, of abstract designs, of flowers, hunters, maidens. The place was as large as Buckingham Palace in London and contained bathrooms with water drainage, ventilating systems, waste chutes, and many of the conveniences of modern times.

On the European continent, most of Greek architecture was colored inside and out, though moist climate over a number of centuries has pretty well obliterated it. The Classical tradition persisted, as in Egypt and Asia Minor. Even in sculpture, where the Greeks far surpassed the artists of other nations, he did not venture to extend the palette. Frederik Poulsen describes Greek coloring:

When the reliefs were discovered, they were richly painted, and still the colors have not all faded. As was indicated in the treatment of the metopes of the Sicyonian Treasury, the background was blue. The figures are treated in blue, green, and red, the last color in two shades, light red and golden-red. The clothes are red with blue borders, while the colors are changed when two or more articles of clothing or armor are worn. The helmets are blue, with red ornamental stripes on the edges, to pick them out from the blue background; the last features remind one of the little red nimbus which in red-figured vases divides the dark hair of the figures from the dark ground. The outsides of the shields are alternately blue and red, their insides red, with a narrow colorless border along the edge, a color scheme answering exactly to that of figures on the Aeginetan pediment. The bodies of Cybele's lions are colorless, but the manes, harness, and yoke are red. The tails and manes of the horses are red, or where several are seen close together, alternately red and blue.

In his *Gods, Graves and Scholars*, C. W. Ceram reports on a similar finding: "The plastic works of the ancient Greeks were gaily colored. Statuary was deeply dyed with garish pigments. The marble figure of a woman found on the Athenian Acropolis was tinctured red, green, blue, and yellow. Quite often statues had red lips, glowing eyes made of precious stones, and even artificial eyelashes."

It was because of such reports that Rodin was said to have struck his breast and shouted, "I feel it here that these were never colored."

But colored they were, all Greek sculpture and all Greek architecture! Yet the expression was better and showed a finer respect for mass and delineation.

On the exterior of the Parthenon, marble was coated with an ivory tint. The colors used for the capitals of columns, for relief sculpture, cornices, and friezes were red, blue, yellow, gold, black. These hues also extended into the interior, and the great statue of Athene was suitably and symbolically hued.

Greek culture was carried to Rome, as were Greek philosophy, political theories, gods, science, and colors. Symbolism began to fade, but only partially. As a matter of fact, there is evidence that a good number of early painters and decorators came from Greece and were put to work because of their knowledge and skill with color. The Romans were builders at heart and made more lavish use of raw materials, marbles in bright hues, gold, bronze, mosaics. The gods, however, were still identified by color. Purple, the imperial color of Rome, was in reality a magenta and was sometimes referred to as red. It traces from Greece and is described by Richard Payne Knight as follows: "The bodies of Roman Consuls and Dictators were painted red during the sacred ceremony of the triumph, and from this custom the imperial purple of later ages is derived." The emperor in his purple (or red) robes, embroidered or spangled with gold, was the personification of Jupiter. His chariot was drawn by white horses. A wreath of laurel was upon his head. His face was reddened with vermilion.

Roman buildings disintegrated, as did Greek. In Etruscan cities such as Tarquinia (ca. 500 B.C.) interior walls were decorated with ivory tints, red oxide, golden ocher, blue, green. Designs were more realistic than in Greece.

Then through one of the world's most heinous catastrophies, history left a most remarkable and lucid record of interior color application.

It was in August of 79 A.D. that Mount Vesuvius in Italy erupted without warning. The top of the mountain split apart, and a flood of volcanic ash, smoke, and lethal gas buried cities and their inhabitants, apparently in an instant.

What seems incredible today is that seventeen hundred years elapsed before Pompeii and Herculaneum were substantially unearthed. Except for the inroads of a few venturesome and haphazard diggers, the civilization lay buried all during the Renaissance itself. Little of what it held was seen by the masters of Italy or Europe. It is rather startling to know that virtually no artists of the Renaissance, painters, muralists, architects, saw the marvels of Pompeii and Herculaneum or even knew much about them. Yet, as the cities lay buried, both Gothic and Renaissance art and architecture flourished and took directions of their own.

It was Johann Winckelmann who first devoted himself to the task of excavation during the middle of the eighteenth century. (A bit of digging had been done previously in 1737.) Soon light of day fell upon architectural splendors, rows of houses, temples, theaters, tablets, papyrus rolls, jewelry, utensils, wall paintings, frescoes, all fresh with color.

The color record of Pompeii and Herculaneum is exceptionally complete. While much freedom of expression was shown, the tradition was still Classical and repeated almost the same colors of Egypt and Greece. There was a bold and uninhibited use of bright colors and deep colors, including black, in large areas and over entire walls — offset by painted decoration and ornament. Typical of Pompeii were wall backgrounds and wall panels in black, vivid green, vermilion red, red oxide, golden orange, golden ocher, azure blue. Decorations, figures, ornaments were in a full palette, a palette as complete and rich as that

employed by designers and decorators today.

It was during the Renaissance, of course, that modern traditions and period styles had their origin, for it was after the Renaissance that Western culture rose out of medieval seclusion and flourished vigorously.

But the Renaissance had to wait for a few intervals of architectural and decorative art.

In the Byzantine style (5th and 6th Centuries A.D.) there was a show of great luxury. St. Sophia's at Constantinople was built with colorful marble in red, green, blue, black. Portals were covered with gold leaf. Jewels and pearls were woven into curtains. There were carved cedar, amber, ivory, mosaic, cast metal. The architecture and the application of color influenced certain later Christian churches and also, indirectly, the mosques of Islam, the Alhambra, and the Alcazar.

With the growth of the Gothic style in the Middle Ages, the more formal and symbolic qualities of ancient times were replaced by naturalistic tendencies. As in Byzantium, color was a stimulus to emotion, not a definition of universal principles.

James Ward has written that the early buildings and monuments of France before the Renaissance were colored inside as well as out. Realistic paintings and decorations were common. The facade of Notre Dame still bears traces of such art. There was much gilding. Describing the great cathedral, Ward writes:

The coloring occurred principally on the moldings, columns, sculptured ornaments and figure work. The outside coloring was much more vivid than the inside work. There were bright reds, crude greens, orange, yellow ochre, blacks and pure whites, but rarely blues, outside, the brilliancy of light allowing a harshness of coloring that would not be tolerable under the diffused light of the interior. The large gables of the transept also bear traces of old painting. There is also evidence that the greater portion of similar edifices of the thirteenth, fourteenth and fifteenth centuries, in France, were decorated in color.

Regarding Notre Dame, the *New York Times* (September 9, 1979) ran a story by John Russell titled "An Eloquent Visitation by Medieval Kings." The report discussed a number of decapitated heads from statues that had stood for more than 500 years on the west façade of Notre Dame, which were exhibited at the Metropolitan Museum in New York. Around 1793, during the French Revolution, the statues were pulled down, broken up, and apparently destroyed. Because Notre Dame was well documented and its art recorded in engravings, replicas of the statues were replaced in the 1840s and 50s. In 1977, with much surprise and delight, 21 of these severed heads were found in the courtyard of a French bank. As Russell reported:

There was high drama in the episode, even so. No one had expected to see these statues again. Even in battered form they have an incomparable power and majesty. Bruised eye sockets, broken noses and broken lips bear, one and all, the lineaments of outrage. Quite apart from that, several of them bear traces of original paint. They give us, therefore, an authentic if much effaced idea of what the west front of Notre Dame must have looked like in the second half of the 13th century. Our century has been haunted by the idea of a time 'when the cathedrals were white'; but the truth is that in the beginning those cathedrals were not white at all, but vivid with high color.

In Mexico and Central and South America, the pyramids and temples of the Mayans and Incas were virtually covered with colored ornaments and exterior wall decoration. The colors were the same as those used elsewhere throughout the ancient world.

In Islamic architecture, however, the use of color was unique. From the 7th to the 12th centuries and later, Islamic culture and religion spread throughout the Near East, into India, across North Africa, and into Spain. Magnificent mosques and palaces, many with bulbous domes, made free use of terracotta, mosaic, tile, and brick. Decorations featured flowers, plants, and geometric patterns.

The Persian Moslems were artists of the first rank. The imperial mosque at Isfahan in Iran, built around 1598 under Shah Abbas, is one of the masterpieces of world architecture. It and other buildings in the city are exquisitely decorated with colorful tiles and mosaics.

What is curious about Islamic architecture is that red is seldom found, despite its prominence in the art of all other ancient civilizations! The mosque at Isfahan and the Blue Mosque in Istanbul glorify blue, turquoise, green, and gold. One wonders about the omission or avoidance of red, perhaps the most human and dynamic of all hues in the spectrum. The explanation is as yet unknown.

When classicism was reborn, following the findings of Johann Winckelmann (c. 1762), Greek revivals spread across the western world—and America—like an epidemic. In America (and in England) the simple beauty of the Georgian style was abandoned in favor of forests of Greek and Roman columns. Every state built its capitol to resemble Greek temples. (It is said that the columns of the Supreme Court Building in Washington rest only on the ground and support nothing. They are there for effect!)

American architecture has become quite austere. With the influence of the Bauhaus, natural materials (such as stone and concrete) were featured. Yet a revival of exterior color is coming, as has been related in Chapter 11.

APPENDIX B

The Colors of Period Styles

Traditional period styles, still revered and repeated these days, trace mainly from the Renaissance. Victor Hugo described the Renaissance as "that setting sun all Europe mistook for dawn." What happened is that while Classical values were reborn, color left the exteriors of buildings to find refuge indoors.

Renaissance buildings and palaces were for the most part designed to feature works of art and are empty without them. Alcoves and niches are made for sculpture, bordered moldings on walls and ceilings for paintings. Everywhere there is a profusion of detail, with empty space virtually unknown. Although the whole mythology and spirit of Christianity dominates the period, its outward religious expression is frankly pagan.

There is little doubt but that the art of oil painting led to a sudden fascination with color. Anything could be done and was done. Yet when Renaissance interior decoration is screened or digested, it contains, for all its luxury, definite echoes from Greece and Rome.

However, if the Classical tradition was still extant during the Renaissance, the artists of the time soon forgot about it and lost themselves to the greatest orgy of color known to history, for out of the Renaissance, out of man's search for personal values, came the Creative tradition, which in principle and spirit still guides cultural expression today.

In differentiating between the Classical and the Creative traditions, the colors that a person might choose for a flag, a crest of some sort, or the class colors of graduation, will be studied for their venerable meanings; the researcher may consult heraldry or the recognized tokens of religious rite or education. Yet the same person choosing colors for the living room of a home will either follow the vogues of fashion or indulge in personal fancies.

Thus in the Classical tradition, the colors are usually simpler and fewer in number. There is a tendency to reduce the complex world of color to precise elements. In the Creative tradition the sky is the limit. There is a tendency to get away from the primary and to seek that which is different, original, exclusive, subtle, sophisticated.

To appreciate the spirit of Renaissance decoration, one should understand that virtually nothing was plain. Interior design would wait a couple of centuries, beyond the Baroque and Rococo styles, for a revival of the Classical tradition and a return to formality and simplicity. Yet in the Renaissance, creative originality in color had its first truly great epoch — the result not only of competent developments in the manufacture of dyestuffs and pigments, but of the personal desires of artists to express inner compulsions, dreams, and insights. Now color would become a highly personal art, and decoration would cater to the boundless domain of taste and emotion as sensed within the human psyche and not as directed by any outside convention or authority, religious or otherwise.

There are many features peculiar to Renaissance decoration. One is a lavish application of gold, not only for ornament but for large areas on which decorations were applied. There is much use of paintings, moldings, pilasters, columns, capitals, cornices, carving, marquetry in imitation of mosaic and inlaid marble. Wall areas may be rich and dark, or off-white, but they are rarely subtle, pastel, or muted. All is extroverted and sensuous, including the spiritual. If the Greeks had a golden age in the philosophical sense, the Italian Renaissance had one in the material sense.

Ivory white and cream were often used for whatever blank spaces might exist or as backgrounds to colorful ornaments. Metallic gold was everywhere. There was no hesitancy in the use of Pompeii Red, Medium Malachite, Green, Golden Ocher, Della Robbia Blue. **The artist discovered that deep hues like cobalt, garnet red, and brown and copper tones made dramatic foils for a full spectrum of pure colors. Spaces were large, life vigorous and outgoing.**

It would take the French and the English to refine the Renaissance, conceive of smaller rooms that required less vividness, and thus introduce those more intimate pastels and muted hues which the world has now come to associate with modern interior decoration.

French interiors prior to the Renaissance were heavily Gothic, although they retained something of an Italian quality. Furniture was bulky and substantial, made of oak and only occasionally decorated with color. Walls were painted white or buff for the most part, and many structural features of wood or stone were left exposed. Historically there were reasons for **the French to be the first of European countries to**

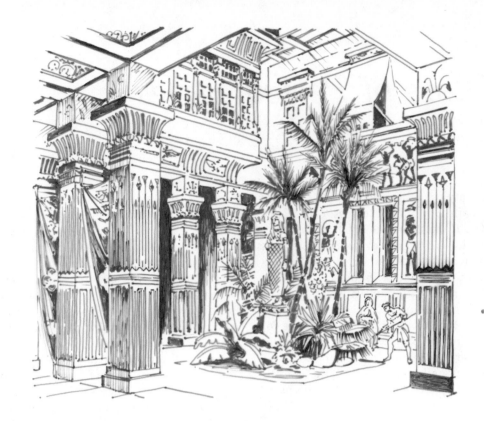

Egyptian interior.

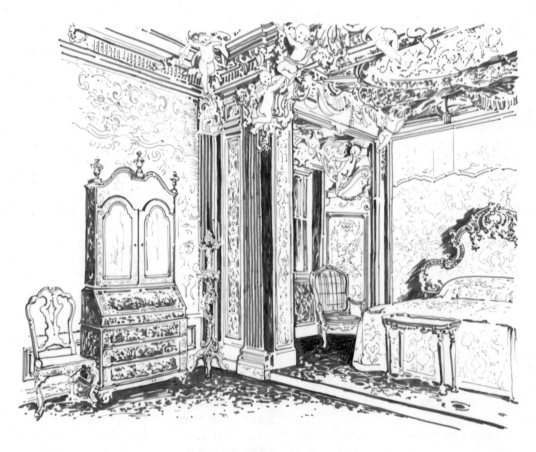

Renaissance interior.

catch the spirit of the Italian Renaissance and to bring its manifestations onto French soil. While the Renaissance was in full flower in Italy the two countries were embroiled in power struggles; Louis XII, who reigned from 1493–1515, fought the Italians at Milan and Genoa but failed at Naples.

His successor, Francis I, one of the truly great kings of France (he reigned from 1515–1547), resumed the Italian wars and developed a respect for the great artists of Italy. To his court came such eminent Italian masters as da Vinci, Cellini, Andrea de Sarto, and one of the famous Della Robbias. There were craftsmen with Italian, German, Flemish, and Spanish backgrounds. Both Fontainebleau and the Louvre were begun. Bulky Gothic ornaments gave way to more delicate motifs, the laurel and acanthus, which planted the seeds of later Baroque and Rococo styles.

Color at the time of Francis I, therefore, was clearly Renaissance. But French taste and an expression individual to French national temperament and culture would soon become evident and would lead to what may justifiably be considered one of the most elegant of all eras in the history of western interior decoration.

France under Francis I saw the fullest development of the Renaissance spirit. Having been properly schooled, the Frenchman now could strike out and prove the high degree of his individuality.

The Fontainebleau of Francis I and Henry IV was second only to Versailles in magnificence. These abodes of kings became national shrines and were refurbished and redecorated through passing generations. At Fontainebleau there was much use of French Gray. It was applied as a foil for decorations which covered virtually all wall space. The palace today contains rooms that echo the taste of later kings and queens, including Marie Antoinette, Napoleon, and Josephine. There are old salons and chambers which later tenants refurnished. Fontainebleau in its own right is definitely Renaissance and has the lavish gilt of the sixteenth and seventeenth centuries.

The French style flourished and began to blossom. Louis XIII, during his reign from 1601–1643, started Versailles as a chateau and introduced parquet floors, rare woods, rich velvets and brocades — and more color.

Then Louis XIV, the Sun King (reigning from 1643–1715), conquered the Renaissance and brought it under French domination, at least in his own country. Under him, Versailles was rebuilt and enlarged. The head of a vain and powerful France, Louis XIV made Versailles the envy of every living ruler of his day. The Baroque style with all its gilt, ornament, mirrors, tapestries, textiles, marbles, woods, paintings, and other decorations, reached its zenith. Many of the colors were strident — crimson, gold, green. There was a vogue for Oriental forms and hues.

Perhaps it can be said that the Louis XIV period, like the Renaissance, was still masculine. It tended to be heavy and bold in scale. In fact, patronage had come largely from men. French decoration would later come under the influence of women — queens and mistresses — and take on more refinement and restraint. However, two commonly used colors of the Louis XIV style, on the refined side, were Rose Beige and Powder Green. The Powder Green in particular was used in large areas as a paint or stain over wood. It has a delicate beauty which the English later copied, took to their hearts, and used.

What is remarkable about French decoration, notably the period of Louis XV, is the display of a taste different from any that had ever been expressed before. It is closer to modern preferences, for it introduces a new and refreshing subtlety of pastels and muted tones which glorify the Creative tradition and give it a more intimate, personal, and cultured sophistication. In fact, it becomes soft-spoken, affectionate, seductive, and feminine.

It is a curious phenomenon of the reign of Louis XV that it also marked a time in western philosophy and thought known as the Age of Enlightenment. While a decadent court was preoccupied with continuous pageantry and dissipation, men like Voltaire and Rousseau (and Paine and Jefferson in America), wrote of democracy and new freedom for men. France, however, surrendered its resources to its royal court and saw the rise of the upper bourgeoisie. The time was one of self-indulgence and extravagance.

But it was a glorious era for color. Where formerly social life was conducted in big spaces and large salons, there were now smaller apartments and boudoirs. If any one thing is typical of the period, it is the chaise longue. Though the trenchant color might be suitable for the grand interiors, it was too impulsive for the smaller parlor, sitting room, or chamber. And so the art of interior decoration saw its truly first and tasteful application of the delicate tint and refined shade or tone.

Dominant here were the superior taste and influence of Madame de Pompadour, mistress of Louis XV for nearly twenty years. Intelligent, literate, musical, political, she was very much in control and stood at the head of all court functions and intrigues.

It was Madame de Pompadour who patronized the great French painters of the day (Boucher, Fragonard, Watteau, Greuze), made Chinese art (Chinoiserie) popular, founded the Sèvres porcelain industry, and supported Aubusson tapestries and carpets. Her wellsprings for color came from these remarkable sources, feminized the art of decoration, and undoubtedly put her name down in history as the most original, talented, and perceptive patron of color since the time of the Renaissance. This lady's taste, intimate and

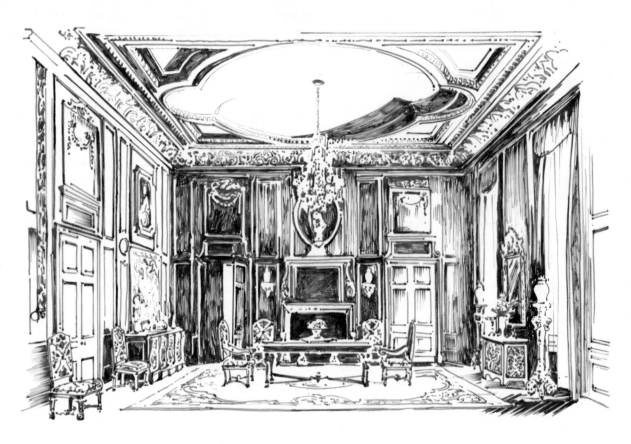

French dining room, Louis XIV period, 1660–1700.

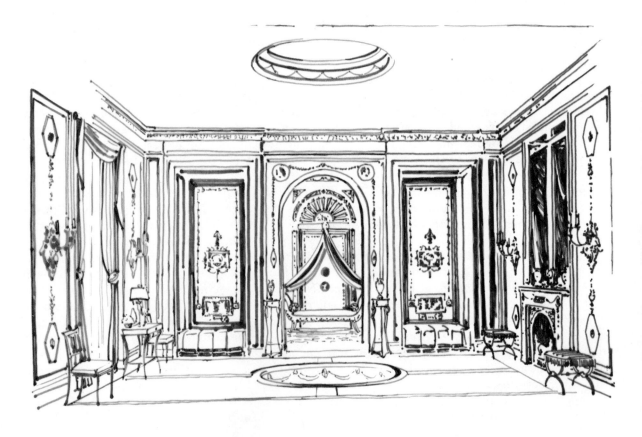

French boudoir, Revolution period, 1793–1804.

personal as it was — and well suited to informal modes of life — has blossomed and reblossomed ever since. There have been few unique or distinct color styles since those of Madame de Pompadour, for it would be difficult to create a "feeling" for color which she did not at one time sense and exploit. The world has emulated her ever since.

New to the art of interior decoration and design were such pastels and lush tones as Powder Pink, Apple Green, French Lilac, Oriental Gold, Sèvres Blue, Rose Pompadour, and Pompadour Blue. Here are the styles which will appear in later decades.

These appealing colors are quite French in character. They were applied to smaller apartments and accompanied by elegant furniture and accessories. A great deal of furniture was painted or gilded. There was much inlay work in wood, marble, porcelain, hand-painted china and metal. Textile and upholstery were florid. One might assume from these interiors that life was a never ending series of games, flirtations, dinners, parties, romps in gardens and woodlands.

Although the form, shape, and plastic character of the Louis XV period was shortly revolutionized, the colors persisted.

By the late eighteenth century French politics stood in dire need of a revolution. The French court had drained the national treasury and gone into debt. As one instance, there was costly intervention by France in the struggle between America and England. Besides, economic conditions had changed. Nobility was being replaced by an upper bourgeoisie, which was making fortunes in industry and trade. This prosperity, however, was not shared with the multitude. Some credit should be given to Louis XVI (he reigned between 1774–1792) for trying to institute reforms, to practice personal economy, and to appoint upright ministers. In this he was quite opposed by his court and by the frivolities and extravagances of his wife, Marie Antoinette.

Revolution was brewing on all sides, although that which took place in interior design and architecture had nothing whatsoever to do with politics. The sharp break that occurred between the Louis XV and Louis XVI decorative styles, and which also occurred in England and America, may be traced to the direct or indirect influence of a German, one Johann Winckelmann. Although Greek and Roman excavations had been going on for some years, it was Winckelmann who truly founded the modern science of archaeology.

Of humble birth, a cobbler's son, Winckelmann was obsessed by a desire to dig into the ruins of antiquity. After a fabulous career he began to publish, between 1762–1767, a series of monumental works on Pompeii and Herculaneum. They immediately astonished and fascinated the world of architecture and decoration and caused the most abrupt change ever encountered in the history of these subjects.

France at the time of Louis XVI went all out, so to speak, for Greece, Rome, and Johann Winckelmann. The feeling tended towards the mathematical and symmetrical, the straight lines rather than curved ones. Although there was plenty of ornamentation, the spirit was Classical.

In matters of color, however, there was serious conflict. There were some who, like the great painter, David, insisted on the pure, formal colors of the Greek and Roman tradition. This was consistent, at least, and was respected in the Directoire and Empire styles that followed. Yet French taste was under feminine domination. Mmes. Pompadour and Du Barry had influenced Louis XV. Now Marie Antoinette, with equal taste, would influence the reign of Louis XVI.

In consequence (and the same is true of England), the Classical tradition set fashions in forms, shapes, and patterns, but the Creative tradition favored the delicate and refined colors unknown to ancient times.

If anything, Marie Antoinette's taste was even more subtle than that of Madame de Pompadour. A few of her preferred tints are Chalk Green, Flesh Pink, Pale Citron.

Following Louis XVI came the Directoire and Consulate Periods which persisted until 1804. Even more that was simple, graceful, and direct was produced in the decorative arts.

With Napoleon and Empire (1804–1815), the revolution went on. Decorative designs, richly and deeply colored, were taken directly from Greece, Rome, and Egypt, lands quite familiar to the conquering Frenchman. Designs showed absolute symmetry, geometric shape, heavy proportion. Many things resembled archaeological findings out of the past. Napoleon designed symbols of his own which included the sphinx, the bee, and the letter N surrounded by a laurel wreath. There were lions and griffins and caryatids. Walls, fabrics, furnishings were full and intense.

Napoleon is said to have liked brilliant colors such as red, Empire Green, Empire Yellow. Empress Josephine, however, had more fastidious taste and preferred smoky tones of gray, blue, mauve, gold, pink.

A few typical French interior color schemes are visualized in Color Plate XIV.

To journey now to England, there is little to relate prior to the Tudor-Elizabethan era (approximately 1509–1603). This marked the end of the medieval and Gothic and the beginning of the Renaissance.

The English take justifiable pride in King Hal and Queen Bess. A lot went on during their reigns — in religious and political upheaval, exploration and colonization, literature, drama, philosophy. Life, however, still clung to medieval precedents. The great medieval hall in which the privileged ate, danced, sang, and often slept, would be relinquished for a more ordered

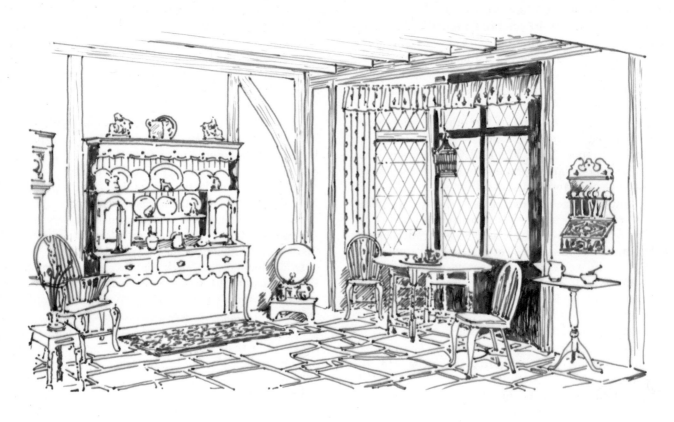

English cottage, 18th century.

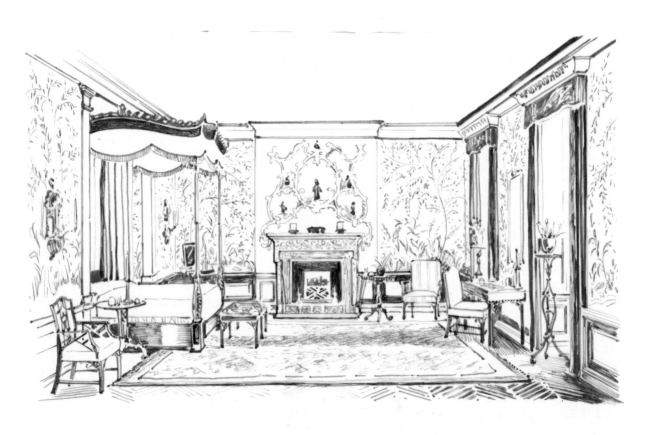

English Georgian, 1760–1775.

and compartmental existence.

Tudor and Elizabethan furniture and decoration were huge, solid, bulky. Walls were mostly oak, stone, brick, and heavy with tapestries. White and buff are perhaps the only colors to be mentioned and may be recalled by the reader in memory of half-timbered Elizabethan structures.

In the Stuart period (1603–1688) which includes Jacobean, Commonwealth, and Restoration, the Renaissance in England reached full bloom. The decorative feeling was massive, solid, and ornate. There were silks, damasks, velvets, brocades, leathers in brilliant hues — plus a new art of lacquering. The colors, however, were still Renaissance and on the bold side.

With the William and Mary, or Queen Anne, period came a more abrupt break which extended from about 1688–1727. King William, in fact, of Dutch origin, did not think much of English taste and set out to change it. Walnut was introduced as a decorative wood and was sometimes bleached. In furniture and decoration, that which had been straight and heavy became curved and convex. Furniture was painted and lacquered, at times in imitation of marble. There was the beginning of an individual English style and feeling, one that was sleek and sophisticated. Chinese wallpaper and porcelain became popular. While there was not much attention to painted walls (decorations were preferred), green was introduced and became the favored color note of the Early Georgian period that immediately followed.

With the Early Georgian style (from 1727 to about 1760), the British really found their own expression. Perhaps no period in all English history is more beautiful, unique, friendly, warm, and intimate than the Georgian. It became the rage in America and is still held in reverence.

The British economy was an influential factor in this development. Up to the eighteenth century there had been strong kings, weak kings, rebels, religious and civil wars. Now there was more diffuse wealth, prosperity in industry and trade. Taste that had flowed into England from Italy, France, the Netherlands, from far-off China, and India, was fused into a definite style having a British quality.

Perhaps climate is an additional factor. Where there is less sunlight, there is likely to be restraint in the use of color. The people who live in colder, foggier, and wetter lands are likely to be sober and diligent; the struggle for shelter and security require greater attention and effort. The home becomes a sanctuary and retreat, and its beauty must be appropriate to its utility.

Much credit for the beauty of the Early Georgian style may be attributed to a series of eminent cabinetmakers and decorators. Foremost among them was Thomas Chippendale II, one of three bearing the famous name. In 1754 he published *The Gentlemen and Cabinetmaker's Directory* which had phenomenal sale and distribution, was the first of many prototypes, and was so wholeheartedly accepted that it set the pattern of English furniture and decoration as if by national law. Seldom has the work of one man been so suddenly and generously adopted.

Thomas Chippendale was quite a genius. A great admirer of both the Louis XIV and Louis XV periods, he did not just abstract what was good from these sources, he amalgamated them along with what he admired from the Italian, Gothic, and Chinese. His was an eclectic talent that founded an enduring "school." There would be Chinese Chippendale, Scottish Chippendale, Irish Chippendale — even Philadelphia Chippendale — as time went on and his imitators became legion.

Chippendale introduced mahogany as a decorative wood. He gave a rich interpretation to other national cultures. There are beautiful furniture pieces, textiles, carpets, mirrors, wallpapers which represent a sort of universal beauty, surprisingly varied, but all with a dominant and consistent English flavor. He was the father of the entire style of the Middle Georgian period. What he designed looked English and was English. Products of his creation swept across his own land and made quite a conquest in America despite political troubles with the American colonies.

Typical Early Georgian colors are Soft Georgian Green, Deep Georgian Green, Georgian Blue, Georgian Gold.

The entire magnificent era of English furniture design and decoration — from Chippendale through Adam, is known as the Georgian. As occurred in France, however, there was a sudden change in the midst of all this creative effort, due in large part to the archaeological findings and writings of Johann Winckelmann on Pompeii and Herculaneum, previously mentioned.

And as in France, while there was an inspired revival of Classical forms, shapes, and designs, the colors became predominantly pastel, as they did at the time of Louis XVI. (In America the same break occurred between the Georgian-Colonial tradition and the Federal. Williamsburg, for example, is Early Georgian, while Mount Vernon is Late Georgian.)

Late Georgian really means the Brothers Adam. Scottish by birth and architects by training, they revolutionized the decorative arts of England. Robert Adam, the best known, visited Italy, was imbued with the Classical spirit, and returned to London to be elected a Fellow of the Royal Society and appointed architect to the King and Queen. He was at one time (1768) a member of Parliament. A partnership with his brother, James, became known as the Adelphi.

Adam was a great innovator. All of his designs were formal, refined, classically pure and true — and perhaps "dry" for all this. If Early Georgian had a livable

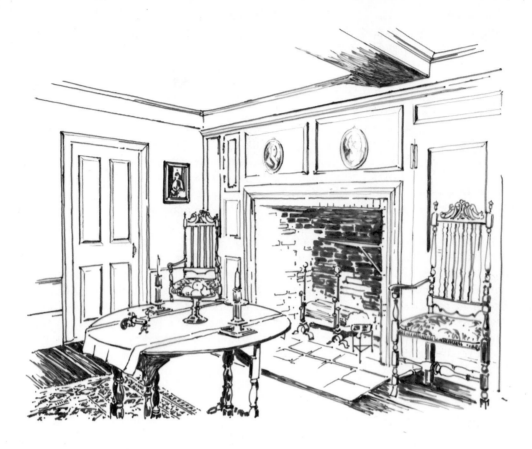

Early American, 1730.

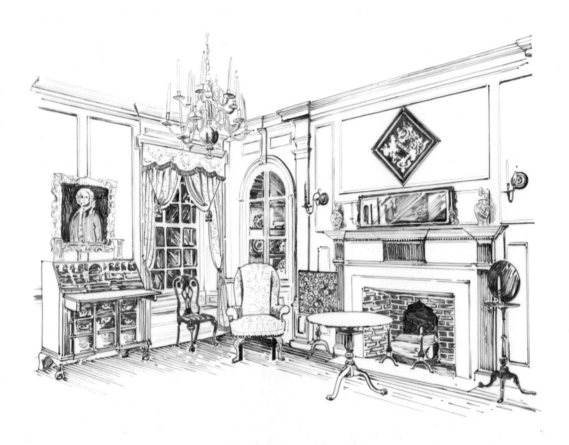

Queen Anne and Chippendale, American, 1750.

and homelike quality, Adam Georgian acquired certain of the stiff elements of a museum.

Adam furniture was quite beautiful in its simple elegance, symmetry, fineness, and squareness. He brought fame to the sideboard with its silver service. His furniture showed restraint and deliberation. There were lighter woods, such as satinwood, much inlay work, slender and delicate ornament. Many home items were gilded. Carving gave way to inlaid and painted designs having cream, pale green, white, or even black grounds. Where the designs were painted, the colors used were also pastel. Nothing was to be officious, aggressive, or pretentious. Oval rooms and rectangular rooms were decorated in pale tints, using paint or silk. Examples are found in Adam Gray, Opal Pink, and Opal Blue.

In perfect harmony with the classicism of Adam was the pottery of Josiah Wedgwood. Grecian ceramic panels or insets were often introduced into cabinets. Wedgwood developed light and deep blue, lilac, and he also used certain Jasper (quartz) colors in red, yellow, green, and brown. At Monticello in Virginia, Thomas Jefferson had a Wedgwood Blue dining room with Wedgwood medallions as ornaments.

With English Regency, the reign of Robert Adam declines. As happened simultaneously to the French Directoire and Empire, English individuality was relinquished for a cold and literal archaeology. The Regency style became grotesque, coarse, and inept. There were Roman couches, bookcases, and cabinets with the facades of ancient temples, stiff elements from Egypt. Besides, the machine age began to predominate over that of the handcraftsman. Colors were preferred dark and heavy, as in France — deep reds, greens, browns. A perfect example of the English Regency style will be found at the Royal Pavilion in Brighton.

A few authentic color schemes for English period interiors are shown on Color Plate XV.

There are a number of unique aspects to the story of color and decoration in America. First of all, there is little to report before the middle of the seventeenth century — and this is a late start as far as history goes. Early settlers brought virtually nothing with them. Once debarked, they were too busy seeking food and shelter to indulge themselves in living accommodations other than log cabins or mud huts.

Then too, settlements were scattered: the English in New England and Virginia, Dutch in New Amsterdam, Swedish in Delaware, German in Pennsylvania, French in Canada and New Orleans, Spanish in Florida, New Mexico, and California.

It was a primitive start with no palaces or chateaux to build or emulate. Architecture began with the simple home, church, and meeting hall. The Renaissance, which had such a pronounced influence in Italy, France, and England, skipped America almost completely. The true beginning was little more than a survival of the Middle Ages and Gothic and quite humble.

Because the American tradition was so strongly influenced by the British, the development of a decorative style constantly reflected that which was English. Much was done from memory. The Pilgrims of New England no doubt recalled the Elizabethan cottages of their birth, while the settlers of Virginia had visions of British architecture, antedating the Georgian.

For functional reasons, however, need was often more significant than desire. Climates were different. There was little time to waste. Many a settler had to build his own edifice. Others had to employ pensioners or laborers, mostly unskilled. Quite important, lumber was everywhere and free for use. As a result, while English taste was commonly expressed, the American colonist very promptly showed skill and originality in adapting it to his materials and to the special demands of his environment. The Cape Cod cottage and salt box home are cases in point. The plantations in Virginia, built on a larger scale and for a different mode of economic life, were more directly British.

So it was that the New England Early Colonial style consisted of timber homes with clay-filled and whitewashed walls — with the fireplace the center of all. The furniture was likely to be Jacobean. Most woodwork, oak and pine, was left unpainted. There were some wall hangings, needlework, pewter. The Pennsylvania Germans, however, used color freely and developed the arts of pottery and glass.

With progress made and the eighteenth century under way, the American Colonial home took beautiful and liveable shape. Walnut became popular as a wood. There was more money to spend. The styles of William and Mary and Queen Anne were introduced. Walls were paneled, and wood trimmings, carved pilasters, and moldings came into use. This promptly led to a reverence for English Early Georgian and for the taste of Thomas Chippendale. Colors soon became rich and full.

Early Georgian, which is so beautifully preserved at Williamsburg, brought glory to the Colonies, and with it wealth and culture. Furniture and furnishings became quite elegant. Walls and woodwork were painted, sometimes in one solid color, sometimes in two different hues. There were different shades of green, soft red, blue, gold, yellow, tan, gray. The Early Georgian manner in America was quite English, for the American colonist was still a loyal, if increasingly disturbed, subject. It was a generation of elegance. Craftsmen on the western side of the Atlantic gained eminence in all the decorative arts. Imports were no longer essential. A certain independence took shape and was to be more clearly defined in the American

Federal period that followed after the revolution.

The colors of American Early Georgian, however, were of brighter, lighter, and cleaner tints than in England — and this is one noticeable difference. Although many of the Williamsburg colors are on the medium and deep side, other Georgian homes in Virginia, Charleston, Philadelphia, Newport favored the pastel. Climate may have had something to do with this, for paler colors are generally preferred in sunny regions.

The Classical revival struck America, just as it did France and England. It is doubtful, however, if the great Johann Winckelmann had much of a direct influence. American revolution was responsible for the Federal style and, at the beginning of the nineteenth century, for Empire taste.

The flourish of Robert Adam in England was during a time when America was far from friendly, hence not much Adam furniture was brought here or made here.

Thomas Jefferson did much to influence American taste in decoration. It is said that the architecture of Williamsburg filled him with scorn, no doubt because of his political memories. As a scholar and capable architect himself, he would restore the Classical ideal, which to him recalled the great republics of Greece and Rome. He designed Monticello and the University of Virginia and, with other designers that followed, reoriented American taste.

For at least fifty years thereafter, the beauty of the Georgian era went into decline — only to come back into favor as its magnificence was seen in true perspective. While Jefferson's classicism still exists in large scale in Washington, D.C., and just about every state capitol, its quality was far too formal, intellectual, and strict for dwellings in which to live a normal life. For such a purpose Georgian was and is more comfortably designed.

In the patriotism of the Federal style, much was drawn from France. There was friendship with Louis XVI and Napoleon. Both George Washington and Thomas Jefferson brought French furniture and taste to America along with French colors. Out of these importations came what is no doubt the most authentic and original of American architectural and interior styles. It entered the White House under Jefferson and was there until the British destroyed it in 1814. (The able restoration of James Monroe, in 1817, brought it closer to French Empire.)

Every region of eastern United States had its Federal examples. There were the magnificent designs of Samuel McIntire in Salem, built from the wealth of sea captains and merchants. There were plantation homes in the south with the air of Italian villas. Eminent, of course, was the Colonial church. In the Federal style the Greek column and pilaster were distinctive marks, together with motifs drawn from eagles, trumpets, thunderbolts, wreaths, etc.

American Federal later shifted toward Empire and got fussier and more archaeological (as it did in French Directoire and Empire and in English Regency). The colors also went from pastels to deeper tones. Then, after 1850, came the Romantic Era which led to Victorianism.

The Georgian colors also apply to America. A few others have been added to them. There is Vernon Gray and Vernon Rose from Washington's home. Washington Gold is the color of the bedroom in which Washington died. There are the Federal colors of the Red Room, Blue Room, and the Green Room at the White House.

See Color Plate XVI for a group of early American interiors.

Victoria was the granddaughter of George III and the niece of the dissipated George IV, who was responsible for Brighton Pavilion and the English Regency style. Her reign lasted for sixty-four years, from 1837–1901. She was queen at eighteen, married her beloved Albert at twenty-one, gave birth to nine children, and became a much bereaved widow at forty-two, living forty years thereafter and dying at the age of eighty-two.

Though Albert was never too popular with the British public, his marriage to Victoria was an idyllic one. He was a wise man, tall, handsome, cultured, and liberal. If the period in which he lived is justly called the Victorian, Albert as Prince Consort was certainly its leading spirit. Elected president of the Society of Arts in 1847, he sponsored a series of exhibits designed to arouse interest in "art manufacturers," which led in 1851 to the Great Exhibit of the Crystal Palace. This exhibit, one of gigantic proportions and influence, spread Victorianism everywhere and was emulated two years later in New York.

The age was distinguished by an endless search for novelty and for pretensions in design, which many persons today still recall. It was supported by machine processes, lathes, and jigsaws, which replaced the craftsmen and led to the most ornate, fussy, and ridiculous fripperies know to history.

If there is a Victorian style, it is any and all things at one and the same time. It is unique because of its conglomeration. Originally begun as a Gothic revival, it went into things Egyptian, Turkish, Moorish, Greek, Byzantine, Persian, Venetian, Chinese, French Baroque, and Rococo. It took ludicrous pride in obelisks, minarets, towers, gables, parapets; in tents, fountains, porches, verandas, pagodas, pavilions; in cast iron fences, vases, deers, and Newfoundland dogs; and it still scars numberless cemeteries with grotesque headstones, monuments, and tombs.

As for the decorative arts of the Victorian Era, some of the furniture was quite attractive and is being reproduced these days. There were chairs and davenports, ottomans, stools, sideboards, tables, beds made of dark mahogany, black walnut, oak, rosewood — not to forget bamboo, the horns of cattle, brass and wrought iron.

These were days of gaslight, a formal and an informal parlor, bay windows, Godey's Lady's Book, Kate Greenaway children, lithographic printing, ornate printing types. Scroll saw decorations, papier-mâché ornaments, stag heads, stuffed birds, flowers under glass, all were in profusion. In the details of the home were beadwork, heavy draperies with tassels and fringe, painted china, embroidered mottoes, needlepoint, decalcomanias, Berlin work, and samplers made from printed designs, cut glass and leaded glass, busts, pedestals, Cashmere and Paisley shawls, gift books and albums, Japanese fans, sea shells, lambrequins, and antimacassars.

Because Albert liked to hunt in Scotland, there was a rage for plaids. Encaustic tile was everywhere and knickknacks were in profusion. Carpets displayed bold patterns in naturalistic motifs and colors. Woodwork came in many deep and lurid finishes. Wallpaper covered walls and ceilings and featured large designs in candent hues. There was much use of marble and of surfaces painted and grained to imitate marble, wood, stone.

There are three highly typical Victorian colors: Perkins Violet, named for the man who discovered coal tar dyes, Victorian Mauve, and Dark Olive. Other intense and heavy colors, of course, were also used, such as vivid red, wine red, rose, brown.

After Victorianism came Art Nouveau, which was quite drab in color. Then came the dull era before World War I, the depressing twenties, World War II, and final emancipation.

Today color is everywhere, free, brilliant, unlimited in choice and application. It has become far more than period, style, fashion. It is part and parcel with modern life, essential to human welfare, indispensable to human environments.

Bibliography

Note. This is a selected list of references, all of which have been important in the writing of this book. Other and minor references have been given in the text.

Babbitt, Edwin D., *The Principles of Light and Color*, University Books, New Hyde Park, N.Y., 1967.

Bayes, Kenneth, *The Therapeutic Effect of Environment on Emotionally Disturbed and Mentally Subnormal Children*, published by author, London, 1967.

Birren, Faber, "The Ophthalmic Aspects of Illumination, Brightness and Color," *Trans. Am. Aca. Ophthalmol. Otolaryngol.* (May–June, 1948).

Birren, Faber, "The Emotional Significance of Color Preference," *Am. J. Occupational Therapy* (March–April, 1952).

Birren, Faber, "The Effects of Color on the Human Organism," *Am. J. Occupational Therapy* (May–June, 1959).

Birren, Faber, *Color Psychology and Color Therapy*, University Books, New Hyde Park, N.Y., 1961.

Birren, Faber, *Color — a Survey in Words and Pictures*, University Books, New Hyde Park, N.Y., 1963.

Birren, Faber, *Color for Interiors*, Whitney Library of Design, New York, 1963.

Birren, Faber, "Color It Color," *Progressive Architecture* (September, 1967).

Birren, Faber, "Psychological Implications of Color and Illumination," *Illum. Engr.* (May, 1969).

Birren, Faber, and Logan, Henry L., "The Agreeable Environment," *Progressive Architecture* (August, 1960).

Bissonnette, T. H., "Experimental Modification of Breeding Cycles in Goats," *Physiol. Zool.* (July, 1941).

Bissonnette, T. H., and Csech, A. G., "Modified Sexual Photoperiodicity in Cottontail Rabbits," *Biol. Bull.* (December, 1939).

Blum, Harold Francis, *Photodynamic Action and Diseases Caused by Light*, Reinhold Publishing Corp., New York, 1941.

Boring, Edwin G., *Sensation and Perception in the History of Experimental Psychology*, D. Appleton-Century Co., New York, 1942.

Burnham, Robert W., Hanes, Randall M., and Bartleson, C. James, *Color: a Guide to Basic Facts and Concepts*, John Wiley & Sons, New York, 1963.

Color and Its Use by the Illuminating Engineer, Illuminating Engineering Society, New York, 1961.

Deutsch, Felix, "Psycho-physical Reactions of the Vascular System to Influence of Light and to Impressions Gained through Light," *Folio Clin. Orientalia* (1937), Vol. 1, Fasc. 3 and 4.

Duggar, Benjamin M. (Ed.), *Biological Effects of Radiation*, McGraw-Hill Book Co., New York, 1936.

Dunlap, Richard, "Probing the Mysteries of Light," *Today's Health* (March, 1963).

Ellinger, E. F., *The Biological Fundamentals of Radiation Therapy*, American Elsevier Publishing Co., New York, 1941.

Ellinger, E. F., *Medical Radiation Biology*, Charles C. Thomas, Springfield, Illinois, 1957.

Evans, Ralph M., *An Introduction to Color*, John Wiley & Sons, New York, 1948.

Gerard, Robert, "Differential Effects of Colored Light on Psychophysiological Functions," Doctoral dissertation, University of California, Los Angeles, 1957.

Gerard, Robert, "Color and Emotional Arousal," *Am. Psychologist* (July, 1958).

Gibson, James J., *The Perception of the Visual World*, Houghton Mifflin Co., Boston, 1950.

Goldstein, Kurt, *The Organism*, American Book Co., New York, 1939.

Goldstein, Kurt, "Some Experimental Observations Concerning the Influence of Color on the Function of the Organism," *Occupational Therapy and Rehabilitation* (June, 1942).

Graham, Clarence H. (Ed.), *Vision and Visual Perception*, John Wiley & Sons, New York, 1965.

Gregory, R. L., *Eye and Brain*, World University Library, New York, 1967.

Harmon, D. B., "Lighting and the Eye," *Illum. Engr.* (September, 1944).

Harmon, D. B., "Lighting and Child Development," *Illum. Engr.* (April, 1945).

Hering, Ewald, *Outlines of a Theory of the Light Sense*, Harvard University Press, Cambridge, Mass., 1964.

Heron, Woodburn, Doane, B. K., and Scott, T. H., "Visual Disturbances After Prolonged Perceptual Isolation," *Can. J. Psychology* (March, 1956).

Hunt, Ridgely, "Miracle of Light," *Chicago Tribune Magazine* (April 28, 1963).

Huxley, Aldous, *The Doors of Perception*, and *Heaven and Hell*, Harper & Row, New York, 1963.

IES Lighting Handbook, Fourth Edition, 1966, Illuminating Engineering Society, New York.

Judd, Deane B., "A Flattery Index for Artificial Illuminants," *Illum. Engr.* (October, 1967).

Judd, Deane B., and Wyszecki, Günter, *Color in Business, Science and Industry*, John Wiley & Sons, New York, 1963.

Katz, David, *The World of Colour*, Kegan Paul, Trench, Trubner & Co., London, 1935.

Katz, David, *Gestalt Psychology*, Ronald Press Co., New York, 1950.

Katz, David, *Animals and Men*, Penguin Books, 1953.

Kelner, A., "Revival by Light," *Sci. Am.* (1951), 184(5).

Klopfer, Bruno, and Kelley, Douglas McG., *The Rorschach Technique*, World Book Co., Yonkers, N.Y., 1946.

Klüver, Heinrich, *Mescal and Mechanisms of Hallucinations*, University of Chicago Press, 1966.

Koffka, Kurt, *Principles of Gestalt Psychology*, Harcourt, Brace & Co., New York, 1935.

Köhler, Wolfgang, *Gestalt Psychology*, Liveright Publishing Corp., New York, 1947.

Kravkov, S. V., "Color Vision and Autonomic Nervous System," *J. Opt. Soc. Am.* (June, 1942).

Kruithof, A. A., "Tubular Fluorescent Lamps," *Philips Tech. Rev.*, Eindhoven, Holland (March, 1941).

Kuhn, Hedwig S., *Industrial Ophthalmology*, C. V. Mosby Co., St. Louis, 1944.

Lazarev, N. M. and Sokolov, M. V., "Ultraviolet Installations of Beneficial Action," report for International Congress on Illumination, Washington, D.C. (1967).

Leiderman, Herbert, Mendelson, Jack H., Wexler, Donald, and Solomon, Philip, Sensory Deprivation, *Arch. Internal Med.* (February, 1958).

Lester, Elenore, "Intermedia: Tune In, Turn On — and Walk Out?" *The New York Times Magazine* (May 12, 1968).

Logan, H. L., "Light for Living," *Illum. Engr.* (March, 1947).

Logan, Henry L., "Color in Seeing," *Illum. Engr.* (August, 1963).

Logan, Henry L., *Amenity Lighting*, Holophane Company, New York, 1965.

Logan, Henry L., *Lighting Research, Its Impact now and Future*, Holophane Company, New York, 1968.

Luckiesh, M., *The Science of Seeing*, D. Van Nostrand Co., New York, 1937.

Luckiesh, M., *Light, Vision and Seeing*, D. Van Nostrand Co., New York, 1944.

"Luminal Color," *Time Magazine* (April 28, 1967).

Maier, N. R.F., and Schneirla, T. C., *Principles of Animal Psychology*, McGraw-Hill Book Co., New York, 1935.

Masters, Robert E. L., and Houston, Jean, *Psychedelic Art*, Grove Press, New York, 1968.

Mosse, Eric P., "Color Therapy," *Occupational Therapy and Rehabilitation* (February, 1942).

Ott, John, *My Ivory Cellar*, Twentieth Century Press, Chicago, 1958.

Ott, John, "Effects of Wavelengths of Light on Physiological Functions of Plants and Animals," *Illum. Engr.* (April, 1967).

Ott, John, "A Revaluation of Ultraviolet as a Vital Part of the Total Spectrum," Obrig Laboratories, Sarasota, Florida, 1968.

Ott, John, "Environmental Effects of Laboratory Lighting," Paper prepared for American Association for Laboratory Animal Science, October, 1968.

Ott, John, "A Rational Analysis of Ultraviolet as a Vital Part of the Light Spectrum Influencing Photobiological Responses," *Optometric Weekly* (September 5, 1968).

Photobiology (March, 1967), reprinted from *Fundamental Nuclear Energy Research*, U.S. Atomic Energy Commission, Washington, D.C.

Pracejus, W. G., *Preliminary Report on a New Approach to Color Acceptance Studies*, General Electric Co., Cleveland, Ohio.

Prescott, Blake Daniels, "The Psychological Analysis of Light and Color," *Occupational Therapy and Rehabilitation* (June, 1942).

"Psychedelic Art," *Life Magazine* (September 9, 1966).

Rickers-Ovsiankina, Maria, "Some Theoretical Considerations Regarding the Rorschach Method," *Rorschach Exchange* (April, 1943).

Rubin, Herbert E., and Katz, Elias, "Auroratone Films for the Treatment of Psychotic Depressions in an Army General Hospital," *J. Clin. Psychology* (October, 1946).

The Science of Color, Committee on Colorimetry, Optical Society of America, Washington, D.C., 1963.

Sheppard, Jr., Joseph J., *Human Color Perception*, American Elsevier Publishing Co., New York, 1968.

Spalding, J. F., Archuleta, R. F., and Holland, L. M., "Influence of the Visible Color Spectrum on Activity in Mice," report of Biomedical Research, Los Alamos Scientific Laboratory, University of California, Los Alamos, New Mexico, 1968.

Tolansky, S., *Optical Illusions*, Macmillan Co., New York, 1964.

Buskirk, C. Van, et al., "The Effect of Different Modalities of Light on the Activation of the EEG," *Clin. Neurophysiology* (1952), 4.

van der Veen, R., and Meijer, G., *Light and Plant Growth*, Philip's Technical Library, Eindhoven, Holland, 1959.

Vavilov, S. I., *The Human Eye and the Sun*, Pergamon Press, London, 1965.

Vernon, M. D., *A Further Study of Visual Perception*, Cambridge University Press, London, 1954.

Vernon, M. D., *The Psychology of Perception*, Penguin Books, 1966.

Walls, G. L., *The Vertebrate Eye*, Cranbook Press, Bloomfield Hills, Mich., 1942.

Werner, Heinz, *Comparative Psychology of Mental Development*, Follett Publishing Co., Chicago, 1948.

Wilman, C. W., *Seeing and Perceiving*, Pergamon Press, London, 1966.

Wolfe, Tom, "The World of LSD," *New York Magazine* (January 29, 1967).

Wright, W. D., *The Rays Are Not Coloured*, Adam Hilger, London, 1967.

Wurtman, Richard J., "Effects of Light and Visual Stimuli on Endocrine Function," *Neuroendocrinology*, Volume 2, 1967.

Wurtman, Richard J., "Biological Implications of Artificial Illumination," National Technical Conference, Illuminating Engineering Society, Phoenix, Arizona, Sept. 8–12, 1968.

Wurtman, Richard J., and Zacharias, Leona, "Blindness: Its Relation to Age of Menarche," Obstetrical and Gynecological Survey, October, 1964.

SUGGESTED ADDITIONAL REFERENCES

Birren, Faber, *Color and Human Response*, Van Nostrand Reinhold, New York, 1978.

Birren, Faber, "Color and Man-Made Environments: The Significance of Light," *Journal American Institute of Architects*, August, 1972.

Birren, Faber, "Color and Man-Made Environments: Reactions of Body and Eye," *Journal American Institute of Architects*, September, 1972.

Birren, Faber, "Color and Man-Made Environments: Reactions of Mind and Emotion," *Journal American Institute of Architecture*, October, 1972.

Birren, Faber, "A Colorful Environment for the Mentally Disturbed," *Art Psychotherapy*, Vol. 1, pp. 255–259, 1973.

Birren, Faber, "Light: What May Be Good for the Body is not Necessarily Good for the Eye," *Lighting Design and Application*, July, 1974.

Birren, Faber, "The 'Off-White Epidemic': A Call for Reconsideration of Color," *Journal American Institute of Architects*, July, 1977.

Birren, Faber, "Color Identification and Nomenclature: A History," *Color Research and Application*, Spring, 1979.

Brown, Barbara B., *New Mind, New Body*, Harper & Row, New York, 1974.

Color, edited by Helen Varley, Knapp Press, Los Angeles, 1980. Foreword by Faber Birren.

R. H. Day, *Human Perception*, John Wiley & Sons, Sydney, Australia, 1969.

Evans, Ralph M., *The Perception of Color*, John Wiley & Sons, New York, 1974.

Faulkner, Waldron, *Architecture and Color*, Wiley-Interscience, New York, 1972.

Gregory, R. L., *The Intelligent Eye*, McGraw-Hill Book Co., New York, 1970.

Halse, Albert, *The Use of Color in Interiors*, McGraw-Hill Book Co., New York, 1978.

Hurvich, Leo M. *Color Vision*, Sinauer Associates, Sunderland, Mass., 1981.

Moss, Thelma, *The Probability of the Impossible*, J. P. Tarcher, Inc., Los Angeles, 1974.

Ott, John, *Health and Light*, Devin-Adair Publishing Co., Greenwich, Conn., 1973.

Porter, Tom and Byron Mikellides, *Color for Architecture*, Van Nostrand Reinhold, New York, 1976.

Rothney, William B., "Rumination and *Spasmus Nutans*," *Hospital Practice*, September, 1964.

Wurtman, Richard, J., "The Effects of Light on the Human Body," *Scientific American*, July, 1975.

Index